The Management of AIDS Patients

Edited by

David Miller
Principal Clinical Psychologist, The Middlesex Hospital, London

Jonathan Weber
Wellcome Research Fellow, Jefferiss Research Wing
St Mary's Hospital, London

John Green
Principal Clinical Psychologist
St Mary's Hospital, London

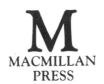

MACMILLAN
PRESS

First published 1986
Reprinted 1986 (twice), 1987 (twice), 1988

Published by
THE MACMILLAN PRESS LTD
Houndmills, Basingstoke, Hampshire RG21 2XS
and London
Companies and representatives
throughout the world

Distributed in North America by
SHERIDAN HOUSE PUBLISHERS
145 Palisade Street, Dobbs Ferry, NY 10522

Printed in Hong Kong

British Library Cataloguing in Publication Data
The Management of AIDS patients.
1. Acquired immune deficiency syndrome-Patients
I. Miller, David   II. Weber, Jonathan
III. Green, John
362.1'9697   RC607.A26
ISBN 0-333-40465-3
ISBN 0-333-40466-1 Pbk

This book is dedicated to all our patients, past and present

H √ H 4096 /14.99 8.91

THE MANAGEMENT OF AIDS PATIENTS

This book is due for return on or before the last date shown below.

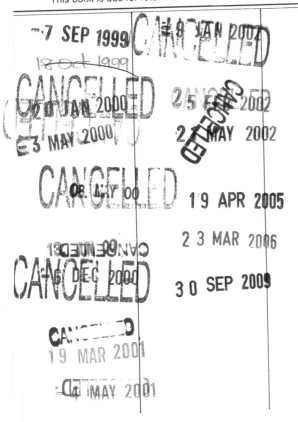
Don Gresswell Ltd., London, N.21   Cat. No. 1208

DG 02242/71

Contents

The Contributors

Greta Forster,
Senior Registrar in
  Venereology
St Mary's Hospital,
Praed Street,
London W2 1PG

John Green,
Principal Clinical Psychologist
and Honorary Lecturer in
Behavioural Sciences,
St Mary's Hospital,
Praed Street,
London W2 1PG

David Houghton,
Research Nurse,
Jefferiss Research Wing,
St Mary's Hospital,
Praed Street,
London W2 1PG

Don Jeffries,
Head of Division of Virology,
St Mary's Hospital,
Praed Street,
London W2 1PG

Elizabeth Jenner,
Senior Nurse,
Infection Control and Research,
St Mary's Hospital,
Praed Street,
London W2 1PG

Peter Kernoff,
Consultant Haematologist and Lecturer
  Haematology,
Royal Free Hospital,
London NW3

Anthony Levi,
Assistant Director Nursing Services,
St Mary's Hospital,
Praed Street,
London W2 1PG

David Miller,
Principal Clinical Psychologist,
The Middlesex Hospital Medical School,
James Pringle House,
London W1N 8AA

Riva Miller
Senior Social Worker/Family Therapist,
Haemophilia Centre,
Royal Free Hospital,
London NW3

Anthony Pinching,
Senior Lecturer and Honorary Consultant
    in Clinical Immunology,
St Mary's Hospital,
Praed Street,
London W2 1PG

Jonathan Weber,
Wellcome Research Fellow,
Honorary Senior Registrar
Jefferiss Research Wing,
St Mary's Hospital,
Praed Street,
London W2 1PG

Foreword

Working in a hospital with a very large clinic devoted to the care of patients with sexually transmitted disease always produced interesting clinical problems. This involved various members of the general hospital staff in a relatively minor way, until the advent of the modern plague due to the AIDS virus. As a physician, I was irresistibly drawn in a very minor capacity as an observer, and soon became aware of the enormous clinical, diagnostic, management and psychological problems engendered by perhaps only one patient, and when these various problems were multiplied by the need to minister to an increasing number, on both an in-patient and an out-patient basis, it was soon apparent that a medical crisis, in relation to both the hospital and the whole community, was upon us. Particularly in a closed institution such as a hospital, the relatively sudden impact of this disease produced sometimes convulsive responses on the part of all members of the staff, and all needed a counselling service, quite apart from that offered to patients and their relatives. Experience on this scale will, it is hoped, be confined to certain centres, but the nature of the disorder is such that all sections of the community need knowledge, so that they may have an informed view, rather than rumour and speculation. This book is produced by a group of workers from different disciplines at St Mary's Hospital and the Royal Free Hospital: I believe it is required reading for anyone who has to deal with the various problems, and to read it is an education into medicine at its most broad in terms of human relationships, and at its most deep in the intricacies of infections and the immune system.

Professor Sir Stanley Peart, MD, FRCP, FRS
Professor of Medicine
St Mary's Hospital, London W2

Preface

Throughout the last 2 years, we have spent a great deal of time in many centres speaking to health staff and managers about the impact of AIDS and HTLV-III infection. This has been in response to the clear need, particularly in those centres sited away from major urban specialist facilities, for information drawn from the more concentrated experience. This information is needed in order to assist the planning of effective management in anticipation of a wider spread of AIDS and related syndromes.

This book does not set out to discuss the more controversial theoretical issues arising from an increasing understanding of HTLV-III infection (although questions relating to the validity of antibody testing and informing the patient of his or her* status are discussed in some sections). Rather, we aim to give details of differing aspects of patient management based on the lessons that have been learnt in recent years. As such, this book provides an integrated, problem-oriented approach to the management of AIDS patients and those with AIDS-related disorders for those who have not yet had such an opportunity to plan and provide large-scale (or even small-scale) treatment strategies.

In doing so we attempt to explain the broad range of implications arising from the context of AIDS for all disciplines that may reasonably expect to play a part in patient management and public health education. The intended readership of the book includes doctors, nurses, laboratory staff and counsellors. Each chapter may be read as a discrete unit, or as part of a whole package. Because it was envisaged from the outset that particular disciplines may confine their perusal to their own specialist chapter, a certain degree of content overlap has been permitted. For those reading all sections, it is hoped that repetition has been constructive, with emphasis having been altered according to the nature of the discipline being addressed.

Because this book is a response to the clearly stated need for practical information on all aspects of patient management, only key references have been provided. References on associated research issues may be gained from those cited here.

*Unless otherwise dictated by context, patients will be referred to in the masculine sense, in order to avoid cumbersome repetition of 'he or she'/'his or her'.

As well as covering the medical and infection control issues, much stress has been placed on the role of counselling in patient management. This is because the counsellor has very important responsibilities in this context: providing essential health education for those at risk; providing essential health information for those who have been diagnosed; co-ordinating post-diagnostic para-medical management; supporting patients, lovers, families and even friends through the various stages of illness. It is hoped that this book itself provides a useful counselling role, in suggesting and reinforcing effective clinical practice in the fight to reverse the spread and impact of this tragic illness.

London, 1985   D. M.

J. W.

J. G.

1

The Clinical Management of AIDS and HTLV-III Infection

Jonathan Weber and Anthony Pinching

INTRODUCTION

In June, 1981, The Centres for Disease Control reported the cases of 5 homosexual men in California who had acquired *Pneumocystis carinii* pneumonia (PCP). In July a further report of 26 cases of PCP and Kaposi's sarcoma in homosexual men in New York was published. All of these patients had a marked impairment of the cellular immune response, with a gross reduction of the T helper phenotype of peripheral blood lymphocytes.

These were the first two reports of the recognition of the Acquired Immune Deficiency Syndrome (AIDS), a disease now known to be caused by an unique new retrovirus, currently called the human T-lymphotropic virus type III (HTLV-III). Similar retroviruses associated with AIDS have been described, and are known as the lymphadenopathy-associated virus (LAV) or the AIDS-related virus (ARV). These three virus isolates are almost certainly identical, and for the purposes of simplicity, the AIDS virus will be referred to as HTLV-III throughout this book.

This infection is transmitted through blood transfusion and through penetrating sexual intercourse, and is now, in the short space of 4 years, epidemic through the Western world and through parts of equatorial Africa. There are now (April 1985) just under 10 000 cases of AIDS in the United States, and 559 cases were reported in Europe by October, 1984. In the United Kingdom 159 cases have been reported. Whereas the early cases of AIDS in Europe were strongly associated with a history of travel to the USA, with homosexual intercourse in New York or San Francisco, latterly most European cases do not report this factor. This intimates that there is now epidemic spread of this virus within homosexual populations in Europe, and certainly within the UK.

The number of AIDS cases in the UK is thankfully small in relation to the USA. However, a significant number of homosexual men are currently infected

1

with this virus in the UK, principally in London, but also in other metropolitan areas. There is therefore a pool of infection which will undoubtedly lead to an increase in reporting of AIDS over the next 5 years. The great majority of the early AIDS cases in the UK have presented initially to STD clinics, or to inner London hospitals. However, latterly an increasing number of patients with AIDS are presenting to their general practitioners, or to district general hospitals throughout the country. While this disease may appear currently to be only of specialist interest, it will be of great importance for general physicians, GPs and all hospital and community workers to have an adequate knowledge of the management of AIDS, as it enters into the differential diagnosis of many common symptoms and signs presenting to virtually all specialities.

The aims of this book are to describe the experience gained at St Mary's Hospital and the Praed St. Clinic in the diagnosis and treatment of AIDS, and other HTLV-III-related disorders. This includes medical, nursing and psychological problems. Our experience is based on the 60 AIDS patients managed here, and on the 600 out-patients with HTLV-III infection who have been studied since 1982.

The great majority of AIDS cases in the UK have been in homosexual men, and this group will be the focus of disease for the foreseeable future. Sexually active homosexual men have a high incidence of all sexually transmitted infections, particularly syphilis, gonorrhoea, peri-anal herpes simplex, wart virus infection and intestinal parasitic infection. It is beyond the scope of this book to deal with the non-AIDS infections in homosexual men, but a bibliography for further reading is included at the end of this chapter.

EPIDEMIOLOGY OF AIDS

AIDS has been reported in sexually active homosexual men; female sexual partners of AIDS patients; children of infected mothers; and persons exposed to blood or blood products, whether by sharing of intravenous needles, by whole blood transfusion or by factor VIII concentrate in haemophiliacs.

Seventy per cent of all cases of AIDS in the USA have occurred in homosexual or bisexual men, and this proportion is greater in the UK, representing the major risk group at present. The cases associated with sexual exposure in Central Africa have been rare in the USA, although this group constitutes up to one-third of all AIDS cases seen in France. It appears that AIDS may be occurring commonly in Zaire, Zambia, Uganda, Rwanda and other equatorial African countries, and these countries must now be seen to represent high prevalence areas for HTLV-III infection; transmission in these areas appears to be through heterosexual intercourse, with an equal number of male and female cases.

This pattern of transmission resembles that of hepatitis B virus infection, with spread through blood and sexual intercourse, and a greater prevalence of infection in homosexual men. AIDS therefore behaves as a sexually transmitted disease.

Table 1.1 Risk groups for acquiring AIDS

Group	Risk activity
Homosexual men	Multiple sexual partners Anal intercourse (active or passive)
Female sexual partners	Vaginal intercourse with infected partner
Children of infected mothers	Transplacental transmission
I.V. drug abusers	Sharing needles/equipment
Haemophiliacs	Pooled blood products (factor VIII)
Blood transfusion recipients	Infected donor blood Usually multiple transfusion
Haitian origin	? Homosexual/heterosexual transmission
Central African origin	Principally heterosexual spread in equatorial African countries

THE CLINICAL MANIFESTATIONS OF AIDS

Introduction

AIDS is a state of immunosuppression caused by the HTLV-III retrovirus. This virus infects a subset of peripheral blood lymphocytes, the T helper cells, which orchestrate many of the functions of the cellular immune system. Infected cells lose their functional capacity, and die prematurely. This defect of cellular immunity leads to susceptibility to infection with opportunist agents, frequently viral, protozoal or fungal in nature. The cellular immune defect also leads to the development of particular groups of tumours, notably Kaposi's sarcoma and non-Hodgkin's lymphoma. These opportunist infections and tumours are similar to those seen in other patients with congenital or acquired defects in cellular immunity. The nature and presentation of these opportunist infections and tumours will be discussed at length below.

It has been increasingly recognised that patients infected with HTLV-III may develop a wide spectrum of other diseases which are not caused by opportunist infection, and which appear to be direct or indirect consequences of virus infection. The commonest of these conditions is persistent generalised lymphadenopathy (PGL); a proportion of patients with PGL (5-25%) will ultimately go on to develop AIDS. The exact relationship between these 'prodromal' disorders and the later emergence of AIDS is still unclear; the majority of PGL patients appear not to progress to frank AIDS in 3–4 years of follow-up. However, the natural history of this disease will not be fully evaluable for a considerable time, owing to the latency of the infection.

The study of HTLV-III infection is in its infancy, and new syndromes are still becoming apparent. The long-term (i.e. > 10 years) consequences of the infection are unknown, but it is reasonable to hypothesise that further neoplastic and other complications may ultimately arise.

Recognition of AIDS

While AIDS is unprecedented, patients with cellular immunodeficiency are not uncommon in medicine. The types of opportunist infection seen in AIDS follow the broad pattern of infections in patients with congenital cellular immune deficiencies (e.g. severe combined immunodeficiency), or with iatrogenic immuno-suppression, as in renal transplantation. Because AIDS causes a specific depletion of the cellular arm of immunity, the infections are predominantly due to viruses, fungi, protozoa and facultative intracellular bacteria. The common feature of opportunist infection is an inability of the host to handle an infecting agent normally. While some of the individual infections may appear bizarre, the pattern of abnormality is predictable in the context of impaired immunity. Thus, in AIDS, patients may have florid persistent ulcerating herpes simplex infection which in a normal host would be a self-limiting vesicular eruption (see Plate 22). Similarly, inability to eliminate mucosal candidiasis is almost universal in AIDS, and plaques of oral candidiasis are a simple biological marker of immuno-deficiency (see Plate 5). AIDS should therefore come to mind when a patient fails to deal normally with infections by agents normally handled by cellular immunity.

Although HTLV-III infection may affect any person in the community through blood or sexual intercourse, the distribution of disease is still largely seen within defined high-risk groups (see Table 1.1). Homosexual men who have anal intercourse with multiple partners are at risk, whereas homosexual men who exclusively have mutual masturbation are at no risk at all. The pattern of sexual behaviour is of great importance, and a detailed account must be elicited. This should include a detailed enquiry into sexual practices (for instance, whether anal intercourse occurs, and whether the active or passive role is adopted) and past history of sexually transmitted diseases. Intravenous drug abusers acquire AIDS through the sharing of contaminated needles and other equipment, and not through abuse of drugs itself. From any patient suspected of AIDS a thorough history of sexual behaviour, drug use, travel to endemic area with intercourse (e.g. to equatorial Africa), or history of multiple blood transfusion must be sought. The travel history is also of considerable importance to the differential diagnosis of opportunist infection, as tropical travel or residence adds the possibility of a wide range of latent tropical infection.

The recognition of an AIDS-related problem therefore comes from the finding of a patient with one of the conditions described below, usually one who fits into the epidemiological pattern (see Table 1.1).

THE CONSEQUENCES OF HTLV-III INFECTION

Figure 1.1 is a schematic representation of the course of HTLV-III infection. Infection may lead to an acute illness associated with sero-conversion. After a latent period, persistent generalised lymphadenopathy (PGL) may develop,

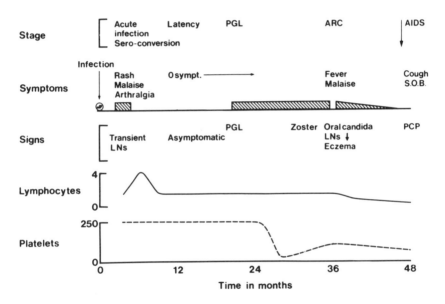

Figure 1.1 Schematic representation of the progression of AIDS

followed by the emergence of debilitating symptoms (the AIDS-related complex — ARC) and finally the development of frank AIDS with opportunist infection. However, it must be stressed that not all patients with AIDS will show these early manifestations, and many patients with PGL or ARC will not develop frank AIDS.

Infection

The HTLV-III virus is present in infected T helper lymphocytes in both an integrated and an unintegrated form. It is probable that the virus is continually budding from the cell surface, leading to a persistent viraemia. The virus can be isolated from semen and saliva, but while the infectivity of semen is possible, there is no evidence that saliva can transmit HTLV-III infection. It has been assumed that the virus is transmitted by transference of small quantities of blood at sexual intercourse. The high likelihood of bleeding at anal intercourse may account for the relative ease of transmission in homosexual men and for the high incidence of infection in men who practise insertion of the forearm into the rectum ('fisting'). Viral transmission may probably occur at both active (penile insertive) and passive (penile receptive) anal intercourse, although epidemiological studies consistently show a greater relative risk with passive intercourse. The occurrence of AIDS in the wives of haemophiliacs and female sexual partners of AIDS patients has demonstrated that vaginal intercourse alone may transmit virus from male to female. Transmission of virus from female to male is suggested epidemiologically but not yet proven virologically. The role of insemination in the transmission of AIDS is uncertain, but as the virus is present in blood and semen, consistent use of barrier methods such as the sheath may reduce transmission. There is no evidence that oral sex may transmit the AIDS virus. This pattern of infection by penetrating sexual intercourse is similar to the transmission of hepatitis B virus infection.

Exposure to HTLV-III by sexual intercourse may not necessarily lead to established infection. Even regular sexual partners of AIDS cases have only a 60% probability of infection as measured by serology. The immunological or virological mechanism for intercourse without infection is not known, but is consistent with that of most other infectious agents.

Acute HTLV-III Infection

After infection, there is an incubation period before the appearance of IgG antibodies. There are now some reports of acute symptoms occurring 4-6 weeks after presumptive infection. In one well-documented case of a nurse infected by finger-prick by a contaminated needle from an AIDS case, a short illness occurred at 42 days after inoculation.

This illness, an acute retroviral infection, is characterised by fever, malaise, headache, flitting arthralgia, maculopapular rash and transient tender lymphadenopathy. In one such case followed at St Mary's, there was a transient lymphocytosis with atypical lymphocytes seen during the viraemic symptoms. Most patients show the rise in T8 lymphocytes typical of the mononucleosis syndrome. The illness resolves in 2-3 weeks, and is associated with the development of non-neutralising IgG antibodies to the P 24 surface glycoprotein of the virus.

While this acute 'glandular fever'-type illness following shortly after infection with HTLV-III undoubtedly has been observed, the majority of patients give no history of illness around the time of sero-conversion. However, any such acute viral illness in a homosexual man should be investigated by viral serology, and HTLV-III is now one of the agents to be excluded.

Latency

Following infection, with or without an acute self-limiting illness, a period of latency follows. During this time it is possible to isolate virus from the peripheral blood lymphocytes by co-culture, and IgG antibody remains positive. The cellular immune system may be entirely normal, in terms of lymphocyte sub-population distribution and absolute number, and the lymphocytes may be functionally normal.

The duration of this latent period is incompletely known. From studies of blood donation leading to transfusion AIDS it has been observed that this period may last for up to 5 years. In homosexual men and intravenous drug abusers this period may be shorter, and it is clear that co-factors may be critical to the period of latency. It seems that the patient may be infectious throughout this time. At present it must be assumed that latency, with infectious virus particles or integrated viral genome present in lymphocytes, may persist for many years and possibly for life.

Persistent Generalised Lymphadenopathy (PGL)

In 1982 Mildvan and others noted that homosexual men at risk for AIDS were developing persistent generalised enlargement of lymph nodes. This condition has subsequently been aetiologically associated with HTLV-III by serology. Follow-up of patients in New York with PGL has shown that up to 25% will develop frank AIDS over a 36 month period; rates of progression in other centres appear to be lower.

A proportion of patients with lymphadenopathy develop further symptoms and signs of HTLV-III infection, such as fevers, night sweats, loss of weight and oral candidiasis. These patients have a higher rate of progression to frank AIDS, and this symptomatic group has been termed the AIDS-related complex (ARC). A proportion of these ARC patients are truly prodromal for AIDS, and will have covert opportunist infection. In others the symptomatology appears to be due to HTLV-III infection alone.

The nomenclature of these groups is confused at present, with different centres referring to clinical syndromes by differing terms. For the purposes of clarity, PGL is used here to refer to those patients with lymphadenopathy alone, in the absence of symptoms, and ARC refers to those with the symptoms and laboratory abnormalities listed in Table 1.4.

It must be stressed that patients with ARC do not necessarily have lympha-denopathy, and indeed the absence of lymph node enlargement in the ARC group may indicate a poorer prognosis.

Definition

PGL is defined epidemiologically by the finding of palpably enlarged lymph nodes of greater than 1 cm in diameter, in at least two or more anatomically distinct sites, lasting for at least 3 months and in the absence of any known cause for lymphadenopathy. Lymph node histology on biopsy usually reveals benign reactive hyperplasia only.

The lymph nodes are readily palpable in the cervical (both anterior and posterior triangles), axillary and inguinal regions, and less commonly in the supraclavicular fossae; epitrochlear lymphadenopathy is rare, and hilar lymph-adenopathy has only been observed in 1% (2/180) cases. The lymph nodes are discrete, non-tender, fully mobile and firm. Marked fluctuations in size may occur over short periods of time, almost on a daily basis. Intercurrent infection may cause dramatic enlargement. The spleen is palpable in 8% of cases, but hepatomegaly is not a feature. The nodes are generally bilateral and remarkably symmetrical. Marked unilateral lymph node enlargement should be an indication for early biopsy. The lymphadenopathy is asymptomatic, and patients may not be aware of the enlargement, which is usually found on examination. The exception to this is occipital node enlargement, which can cause aching discomfort in the neck.

It is important to note that isolated inguinal lymphadenopathy is a common finding in the general population, but particularly in any sexually active male with more than one sexual partner. The finding of isolated inguinal nodes should prompt a search for sexually transmitted infection in the urethra or rectum, particularly for herpes simplex, early syphilis and rarely lymphogranuloma venereum infection.

PGL may be complicated by haematological abnormality, skin rashes and leucoplakia of the tongue. The haematological changes include a lower mean total white cell count, lower lymphocyte numbers and lower platelet numbers. The thrombocytopenia will be discussed below, as up to 10% of PGL patients show a slight or moderate reduction in platelet count during the course of PGL.

Diagnosis

The diagnosis of PGL is made by the clinical findings and the exclusion of the possible differential diagnoses (see Table 1.2). Latterly, the finding of a positive antibody to HTLV-III may assist in the diagnosis of PGL, but it must be stressed that even in the presence of HTLV-III antibody (which is likely to become increasingly prevalent in high-risk groups) other causes of PGL must be excluded — in particular, secondary syphilis and acute Epstein–Barr virus infection. In addition, a small proportion of patients who are infected by HTLV-III and develop PGL may be sero-negative. Table 1.2 shows the differential diagnosis of PGL, with a list of confirmatory tests for each diagnosis.

The role of lymph node biopsy and histological examination of tissue for the diagnosis of PGL is still the subject of debate. This is related to the lack of a pathognomic histological pattern in lymph nodes showing benign reactive hyper-plasia. In uncomplicated PGL, with bilateral, symmetrical nodes and positive HTLV-III serology, it may be sufficient to establish the diagnosis on clinical grounds alone. However, it is necessary to exclude mycobacterial or fungal

Table 1.2 Differential diagnosis of PGL

Diagnosis	Investigations
Secondary syphilis	Examine for chancre, rash, alopecia, etc. Test TPHA, FTA, VDRL Dark-ground examination of suspicious lesions Re-test serology at 4/8 weeks as necessary
Infectious mononucleosis	Marked sore throat with exudate Frequently with tender lymphadenopathy Positive Paul-Bunnell (atypical lymphocytes) EBV/CMV serology if Paul-Bunnell-negative
Acute hepatitis	HAV, HBV, CMV, EBV serology Transaminase titre ? Non-A, non-B hepatitis LNs should not persist > 3 months
Acute toxoplasmosis	Toxoplasma serology for 4-fold rise
Sarcoidosis	Examine for iritis, arthritis, skin lesions Hilar lymphadenopathy rare in PGL Ethnic origin Lack of appropriate risk factors
Brucellosis	Serological tests Occupational/rural exposure
Lymphoma/Kaposi's sarcoma	Biopsy (see also Table 1.16)

infection, lymphoma or Kaposi's sarcoma of the lymph node in atypical presentations (see also Table 1.15). These include patients with grossly asymmetrical or isolated large lymph node enlargement, or in whom matted or fixed nodes are palpable. It is undoubtedly the counsel of perfection to perform a biopsy on every case of PGL, but with increasing clinical experience it does become possible to make a clinical diagnosis, and reserve biopsy for all atypical cases. All lymph node biopsies should be performed on extra-inguinal lymph nodes, owing to the high prevalence of benign inguinal lymphadenopathy in a healthy population.

The histological appearances of PGL lymph nodes reveal in the majority of cases a hyperplasia of the germinal centres, with preserved architecture of the lymph node. However, a proportion of nodes show regression or involution of follicular structure, with ghost-like germinal centres. A smaller proportion will show marked lymphocyte depletion. These latter histological patterns are associated with a greater chance of progression to AIDS over a prolonged follow-up period.

Immunohistology

The examination of frozen sections of lymph node by monoclonal antibody panels enables the distribution of the lymphocyte sub-sets to be assessed. In benign lymph node hyperplasia (e.g. tonsillitis) there is hyperplasia of the germinal centres, with essentially normal distribution of cells being maintained — that is, B cells being within the centre, and T cells in the surrounding interfollicular area. Immunohistology of the lymph nodes in PGL reveals two patterns. In one form there is good preservation of the nodal structure and follicular dendritic reticulum (FDR) cells. The other form shows destruction of the FDR architecture of the germinal centre, with invasion of the B cell areas by T8 lymphocytes; when most advanced, this latter form will be seen on histology as follicular involution. This latter form seems to be associated with a greater chance of progression to AIDS.

Complications

Thrombocytopenia   In our longitudinal study of 180 homosexual men with PGL, 10% developed thrombocytopenia over an 18 month period, defined as a reduction of platelets below $150\,000 \times 10^9/1$ (2 SD). Six of these lowered the platelet count to below $40\,000 \times 10^9/1$, and 4 developed purpura. The remainder demonstrated a lowering of the circulating platelets to approximately $100\,000 \times 10^9/1$, with a gradual rise to normalcy over a 3 month period. It may be possible that this transient drop in platelets is a common phenomenon in HTLV-III infection.

The mechanism of the thrombocytopenia is mediated through immune complex deposition on the platelet surface, with enhanced elimination of platelets through the spleen. The bone marrow reveals an excess of megakaryocytes. This mechanism differs from classical idiopathic thrombocytopenic purpura, where antiplatelet antibodies can often be demonstrated. It remains possible that the majority of patients with PGL may have transient fluctuations in platelet numbers due to alterations in antigen/antibody titres at different stages of infection with HTLV-III.

Six of 180 (3%) of PGL patients have developed thrombocytopenic purpura, in one case prior to the development of PGL. Four of these patients with purpura resolved spontaneously, with a rise in platelet count to $> 100 \times 10^9/1$, while the others required gamma-globulin and, in one case, steroid treatment. However, it is likely that corticosteroid use in this group increases the risk of opportunist infection, and this line of therapy should be avoided if possible. It appears that the thrombocytopenia associated with PGL is generally mild and self-limiting.

Skin Rash   There is an increased incidence of eczema and facial folliculitis in patients with PGL (see Plates 23 and 24). These skin diseases are common in the general population, but are particularly prominent in the context of PGL, and may arise in patients with no prior history of skin disease or atopy of any sort. The eczema is seborrhoeic in distribution; is prominent on the face and chest, particularly in the nasolabial folds and on the forehead; and frequently produces deep cracking of the skin in skin folds. The folliculitis is seen in the beard area and is exacerbated by shaving; no specific organism appears to be responsible for these skin manifestations, although it is common to find *Pityrosporum* fungal spores in association with the eczematous lesions.

Herpes (varicella) zoster has been noticed to occur commonly in patients with PGL. These attacks may be severe, and multidermatome in distribution. The occurrence of herpes zoster is undoubtedly related to minor immunosuppression by HTLV-III, although laboratory studies of immune function may appear normal. Herpes zoster is not seen in frank AIDS. The appearance of herpes zoster may precede the development of opportunist infection by many months, and may be a poor prognostic sign in patients with PGL.

Oral Hairy Leucoplakia   Greenspan recently reported that the white lesions on the lateral borders and underside of the tongue in men with PGL were not caused by candidiasis, as had been presumed, but by a wart virus infection leading to leucoplakia (see Plate 7). Histology of these plaques of leucoplakia reveals the koilocytosis typical of the human papilloma virus (HPV), and electron microscopy reveals particles of Epstein-Barr virus within the lesions. The lesions have characteristic whorls of keratin, giving a 'hairy' appearance. This lesion seems to be unique to HTLV-III-infected patients.

The natural history of this lesion is unknown, but in our experience spontaneous regression may occur. While the optimal treatment of this lesion is unknown, much will depend on the consequences of leucoplakia. Squamous carcinoma of the tongue is reported to be increasing in incidence in young men in New York, over the past 5 years. It is possible that wart-virus-associated leucoplakia may be a premalignant lesion, leading to squamous tumour (as in the cervix uteri).

Leucoplakia of this type must be distinguished clinically from the plaques of oral candidiasis (see Plate 5). *Candida* may infect any part of the oral cavity, but

Table 1.3   Management of PGL

---

(1)   Exclude differential diagnosis (see Table 1.2)
(2)   Biopsy any atypical lymph nodes (see text)
(3)   Confirm aetiology by HTLV-III serology (if in doubt)
(4)   Follow 3-monthly with careful history and examination
(5)   Follow complicated patients (e.g. thrombocytopenia) 1-monthly, or more frequently as required
(6)   Follow FBC, differential and platelet count
(7)   Estimate T lymphocyte sub-sets if total lymphocytes equivocal

---

is also prominent on the underside of the tongue. The lesions of *Candida* are easily dislodged on examination, unlike the fixed leucoplakia. Fungal culture or direct examination of wet preparations for fungal hyphae is a rapid way to make a diagnosis of candidiasis. This is discussed in greater detail in the next section.

The AIDS-related Complex (ARC)

ARC is best defined as symptomatic infection with HTLV-III in the absence of opportunist infection or tumour. It is described as a combination of symptoms, signs and laboratory abnormalities (Table 1.4). The importance of this separate classification of PGL and ARC is due to the differing prognoses between the

Table 1.4   Features of ARC

Symptoms	Severe malaise, fatigue, lethargy
	Loss of more than 10% body weight
	Unexplained diarrhoea for more than 1 month
	Fevers and/or night sweats
Signs	Oral candidiasis
	Oral leucoplakia
	Persistent generalised lymphadenopathy
	Splenomegaly
	Eczema/folliculitis
Laboratory abnormalities	Lymphopenia ($< 1.5 \times 10^9/l$)
	Thrombocytopenia ($< 150 \times 10^9/l$)
	T helper depletion ($< 0.40 \times 10^9/l$)
	Decreased lymphocyte mitogen responses
	Anergy to 3 recall antigens

NOTES
(1) To fulfil the diagnosis of ARC, the patient requires one symptom, one sign and one laboratory abnormality.
(2) Lymphadenopathy is not a prerequisite for the diagnosis of ARC.
(3) The critical aspect of the diagnosis of ARC is to exclude covert infection with any of the opportunist pathogens associated with AIDS (see Table 1.5).

relatively benign PGL (to date) and the higher chance of progression to AIDS in patients with ARC (approximately 25% at 36 months); in addition, patients may have ARC without lymphadenopathy (see definition of ARC, Table 1.4). The poor prognosis of ARC has led to the suggestion that the symptoms are caused by covert opportunist infection, which is not detectable clinically; the prodromal nature of ARC will be further elucidated in the future.

Diagnosis

The diagnosis of ARC can only be made by the exclusion of active opportunist infection or tumour. The symptomatology will direct investigation, and the manner of investigation should follow that laid down in the section on AIDS. The investigation of diarrhoea in ARC, for example, must begin by the exclusion of all the organisms and tumours which are associated with diarrhoea in AIDS. The exact mechanism of the clinical manifestations in ARC is not certain, and it may be found that thorough investigation will uncover covert infection.

The most difficult area of investigation is that of the patient with ARC presenting with fevers, night sweats, weight loss and malaise, with no localising signs. This condition may be debilitating, and multiple investigations may yield no real diagnostic clues. Repeated blood cultures for bacterial, fungal and viral infection should be undertaken, and a thorough investigation of the chest and gastro-intestinal tract. CT scanning of the brain will exclude intracranial abscess or lymphoma. A thorough search should be made for cytomegalovirus (CMV) infection, including culture of the peripheral blood buffy layer leucocytes to exclude CMV viraemia.

ARC may be a debilitating disease, and the balance between extensive investigation of a pyrexia of unknown origin (PUO) and the acceptance of HTLV-III infection as the only discernible diagnosis represents a difficult clinical decision. Patients with PUO in the context of ARC must be followed vigilantly, and any new development of localising signs or symptoms is cause for re-investigation.

PRESENTATION OF AIDS

The great majority of the clinical problems in AIDS arise through cellular immunodeficiency, which results in the development of opportunist infection and tumours (see Table 1.5). These opportunist infections and tumours are of types typically seen in patients with other cellular immunodeficiencies. The organisms seen are largely dependent on the host, and on his prior and present exposure to microbial agents; geographical differences are seen, and prior exposure to sexually transmitted infections may affect the presentation of AIDS in patients in different risk groups.

The commonest infection is *Pneumocystis carinii* pneumonia, which accounts for 50% of all first presentations with AIDS. Over 70% of chest infection in AIDS is caused by this organism, and it may occur at any stage of progression of AIDS. A further 25% of patients will present with Kaposi's sarcoma (KS), with another 10% developing this tumour after initial presentation with an opportunist infection. Other important sites of infection lie in the gastro-intestinal system, the central nervous system and the skin. These will be covered at length below.

Table 1.5   Opportunist infections and tumours of AIDS in the UK

	Common	Uncommon
Viral:	Herpes simplex Cytomegalovirus	Varicella zoster Polyoma virus (JC/BK)
Bacterial:	*Salmonella typhimurium* *Mycobacterium tuberculosis* *M. xenopi/kansasii*	*M. avium-intracellulare* *Legionella* spp.
Fungal:	*Candida albicans* *Cryptococcus neoformans* *Tinea* spp.	*Histoplasma capsulatum*
Parasitic:	*Pneumocystis carinii* *Toxoplasma gondii* *Cryptosporidium* spp.	*Isospora* spp.
Neoplastic:	Kaposi's sarcoma	Non-Hodgkin's lymphoma ? Squamous carcinoma

Pulmonary Presentation

The chest is the most common site of infection in AIDS, and an accurate diagnostic approach to chest disease is an essential basis to the management of AIDS patients (Table 1.6).

Table 1.6   Presentation of chest disease in AIDS

Symptoms	Shortness of breath on exertion Persistent non-productive cough Fever Mild pleuritic chest pain
Signs	May be none Increased respiratory rate Cyanosis (central) Oral candidiasis or other stigmata of AIDS Auscultation generally normal Crackles at lung bases may be present Pleural effusion rare
Organisms	*Pneumocystis carinii* Cytomegalovirus Mycobacteria (including atypicals) *Candida albicans* Kaposi's sarcoma Others rarely (e.g. *Cryptococcus*, *Histoplasma*) Idiopathic lymphocytic pneumonitis (? EBV)

Pneumocystis carinii Pneumonia (PCP)

PCP is the most common infectious problem in AIDS, and is the major differential diagnosis for any diffuse pulmonary infiltrate in the context of AIDS. The patients usually present with a gradual history of increasing dyspnoea with a dry cough. The history may be as long as several months, but is generally 2–6 weeks. A smaller number of patients will present with a more acute history of less than 2 weeks, with florid infections. The variation is undoubtedly related to the degree of immunosuppression of the patient at presentation.

Thirty per cent of patients have had mild pleuritic central chest pains, and most complain of inability to take a full inspiration owing to provocation of coughing and pain. There is always a low-grade fever, often with spiking in the early evening, and night sweats. Examination may reveal no abnormality except increased respiratory rate, but other stigmata of AIDS should be carefully sought, particularly oral candidiasis, plaques of Kaposi's sarcoma, leucoplakia, etc.

The chest X-ray appearances of PCP are characteristic, with a perihilar haze as the earliest manifestation, progressing to diffuse shadowing of the mid- and lower zones, with sparing of the supradiaphragmatic regions until late in the disease (see Plate 1). The shadowing is generally symmetrical, and pleural effusions are rarely seen; air bronchograms may be seen in the lower zones. However, it is important to note that the chest X-ray may be normal in the early stages of PCP; it must be presumed that the immune deficiency delays the appearance of an inflammatory response, and, hence, extensive pulmonary infection may be present with minimal signs clinically or on X-ray.

The investigation of choice for the diagnosis of PCP is a fibre optic bronchoscopy (FOB) with transbronchial biopsy (TBB) of alveolar tissue (see Table 1.7).

Table 1.7   Indications for bronchoscopy (FOB). Any two persisting abnormalities should lead to investigation

Diffuse shadowing on chest X-ray
Hypoxia – p_{O_2} < 80 mmHg
Persisting pulmonary symptoms
Reduced Tl_{CO} with preserved spirometry (< 70% predicted)
Abnormal gallium lung scan

In addition, broncho-alveolar lavage (BAL) will enable cytological examination of alveolar washings, and, hence, a rapid result (see Plate 2). The transbronchial specimen may also be impressed onto a glass slide and immediately fixed in alcohol (a 'touch' preparation) for early cytological assessment. The diagnostic approach using FOB will result in a diagnosis in the majority of cases (see Table 1.8). The failure to make a diagnosis in presenting chest infection will result in confusion and diagnostic uncertainty. We would recommend that a strenuous

Table 1.8   Examination of specimens from FOB

TBB:	Histology (formal saline) — stain for PCP/acid-fast bacilli (Plate 2)
	Virology (viral transport medium) — culture for CMV
	'Touch' prep. for cytology
BAL:	Microbiology — Gram stain and culture: bacterial
	fungal
	ZN stain L–J slope
	Viral culture for CMV
	Cytology of lavage fluid

TBB = trans-bronchial biopsy; BAL = broncho-alveolar lavage.

attempt be made to make an accurate diagnosis in all cases of chest infection in AIDS, unless the concurrent infections of the patient make this approach hazardous. There is no place for empirical therapy in AIDS at this time.

The necessity for an accurate diagnosis in AIDS pneumonia is threefold. First, there may be multiple infections present in the lung, all of which may be fully treatable. Second, the diagnosis of AIDS is a clinical one, and involves the finding of an opportunist infection; a patient with or without HTLV-III antibody may still develop typical or atypical pneumonias, without association with AIDS. Failure to perform bronchoscopy will result in inability to make a diagnosis of AIDS, and therefore no prognostic information can be given to the patient. Third, the decision to ventilate a patient with respiratory failure cannot be taken without an attempt at diagnosis.

The specimens from bronchoscopy should be examined histologically, bacteriologically, virologically and by cytology. Cytological examination, in particular, enables a speedy diagnosis to be made after the collection of samples.

Differential Diagnosis of PCP

Cytomegalovirus (CMV) It is common to culture CMV from the lung biopsies of patients with PCP, and CMV is a common finding from many sites in patients with AIDS. However, it may also be a primary pathogen of the lung, presenting with an atypical pneumonia clinically indistinguishable from PCP, although the history may be shorter than with PCP. The chest X-ray appearances may be similar, although reticular shadowing extending to the periphery of the lung fields is more typical of CMV. Diagnosis is by TBB lung biopsy for histology, and BAL with a positive viral culture for CMV in fibroblast cell lines.

Mycobacterium spp. Atypical mycobacteria, especially *Mycobacterium avium intra-cellulare* (MAI) have been a significant clinical problem in the USA.

While this species has been rare in the UK, owing perhaps to differences in geographical distribution of the organism, increasing numbers of *M. tuberculosis* and *M. xenopi/kansasii* infections are being seen. As there is little cellular response to mycobacteria in AIDS, the organisms are plentiful in tissue, but the clinical signs may be few, and there may be no chest X-ray abnormalities. At present, diagnosis of mycobacterial infection is slow, and treatment of the atypical organisms is largely unsuccessful. *M. tuberculosis* is a high-grade pathogen, and appears as a clinical infection early in AIDS, when some cellular response may be preserved (e.g. positive Mantoux test); the atypical mycobacteria are low-grade pathogens, and are seen in AIDS as late or preterminal infections, with minimal cellular response and large numbers of visible organisms.

Candida albicans Invasive candidiasis is a common event in AIDS, and generally confined to the gastro-intestinal tract. However, invasive candidal pneumonitis has been seen on rare occasions, presenting as an acute chest infection, with rapid opacification of the mid- and lower zones on chest X-ray, and severe hypoxia (see Plate 4). Diagnosis is made by culture of BAL fluid, and by cytology of the lavage cells showing *Candida* within alveolar macrophages.

Kaposi's Sarcoma KS may affect any internal organ except the brain. Pulmonary KS may present with chest X-ray abnormalities and hypoxia. Fever is less common with KS than with PCP, and the chest X-ray signs are more likely to be unilateral or nodular than diffuse; pleural infiltration by KS may present with unilateral pleural effusion. The diagnosis is difficult to make through TBB, although plaques of KS on the bronchial mucosa may be seen at bronchoscopy. Investigation of pleural effusion should include pleural biopsy to search for KS. Post-mortem examination suggests that pulmonary KS may be relatively common in patients with cutaneous disease, but that the proportion of patients with symptoms is small.

Treatment of PCP The treatment of PCP with co-trimoxazole is effective, and initial therapy with an intravenous regimen appears to be well tolerated and led to defervescence in 3-5 days, with radiological resolution in 14-21 days. However, a proportion of patients with overwhelming infection will die in the first attack, regardless of therapy. The survival per episode of PCP is improving, largely owing to prompt diagnosis and treatment. The early recognition of what may be subtle symptoms or signs as an indication for bronchoscopy may be the major factor in improving the survival per episode of PCP.

Co-trimoxazole will cause a maculopapular drug rash in up to 80% of patients in AIDS at about 8-12 days, irrespective of preceding sulphonamide allergy (see Plate 3). If this rash does not involve the mucosal surfaces, it may be possible to continue treatment through this adverse reaction, and the rash should subside in 3-5 days. Sometimes halving the dose of sulphonamide is helpful in reducing symptoms, without jeopardising treatment. Severe skin reactions will necessitate

Table 1.9 Treatment of chest infection in AIDS

Organism	Diagnosis	Treatment	Adverse effects
PCP	FOB/TBB	Co-trimoxazole i.v. 1.92 g/24 h Oral 16 tabs/d for 21 days	Rash (80%) Leucopenia Thrombocytopenia
		Pentamidine i.m. 4 mg/kg	Hepatotoxic Hypotension Hypoglycaemia Muscle abscess
		? Dapsone/ ? Trimethoprim	
CMV	FOB/BAL	DHPG i.v. Foscarnet i.v. 0.08 mg kg^{-1} min^{-1}	? Bone deposition
Candida	FOB/BAL	Amphotericin i.v. 1 mg kg^{-1} day^{-1} 5-Flucytosine p.o. 2-2.5 g q.d.s.	Renal, hepatotoxic, rigors Cytopenia
Mycobacterium avium intra-cellulare/xenopi/ kansasii	Sputum/FOB/BAL	Quad. therapy ? Ansamycin ? Clofazamine	As for drugs used

a change in therapy to pentamidine or dapsone, as will severe neutropenia or thrombocytopenia, if these are resistant to folinic acid.

There is no cumulative benefit from combining co-trimoxazole and pentamidine. The efficacy of dapsone with or without trimethoprim has yet to be fully assessed, but it appears that a dapsone/trimethoprim combination is effective and causes fewer side-effects.

Our experience to date has shown that recurrence of PCP after effective treatment for 3 weeks is rare, and, hence, we do not currently use anti-PCP prophylaxis after a single episode of PCP. It has been suggested that Fansidar (pyrimethamine/sulphadoxine), 1 tablet/week, may be effective as prophylaxis, with little apparent problem from adverse reaction. Prophylactic Fansidar should certainly be considered for any patient with a proven recurrence of PCP.

Prognosis It has been reported that the mean survival after one episode of PCP is only 28 weeks, and that 2 year survival after one episode of PCP is zero. These figures may be unduly pessimistic, as they reflect experience with the early and most florid AIDS cases. Early diagnosis and prompt treatment may well prolong life expectancy, and our experience shows that responders may be expected to have a mean of 8 months infection-free (range 2–18 months) to date. However, survival over 2 years from diagnosis of opportunist infection in AIDS would appear to be rare.

Gastro-intestinal Presentation

The presentation of gastro-intestinal infection or tumour in AIDS is remarkably non-specific (see Table 1.10). The symptoms are usually those of diarrhoea and loss of weight, whatever the site or type of infection. Frequently the clinical signs may be absent or minimal, and diagnosis is therefore by a thorough knowledge

Table 1.10 Gastro-intestinal infection in AIDS

Symptoms	Persistent diarrhoea for > 4 weeks – either profuse watery stool or 4–5 formed stools/day; mucus rectal discharge common; bleeding rare Colicky abdominal pains + distension Loss of > 10% body weight Dysphagia Peri-anal discomfort/ulceration ('piles')
Signs	Oral lesions: leucoplakia candidal plaques KS lesions Abdominal tenderness/rebound Lymphadenopathy/splenomegaly Cachexia Peri-anal ulceration (herpes simplex) Occasional tender hepatomegaly
Organisms	*Candida* oral/oesophageal *Salmonella typhimurium* (+ other spp.) *Shigella* spp. Herpes simplex proctitis CMV colitis Cryptosporidiosis/isosporosis KS of the gut

of the likely pathogens and a thorough search for them with the appropriate bacteriological techniques.

The diagnostic problem in approaching gut disease in AIDS is to distinguish those patients with the gastro-intestinal symptoms of ARC (diarrhoea, loss of weight; see Table 1.4) from those patients with AIDS and infectious causes for the symptoms. An ordered approach to include all possible pathogens will result in the appropriate diagnosis.

Specific Presentations

Candida spp. *Candida albicans* is a ubiquitous infection in AIDS and may colonise any part of the gastro-intestinal tract, from the mouth to the anus. The most common site of infection is the mouth and oropharynx, and oral candidiasis is the hallmark of the prodromal stage, the AIDS-related complex (ARC). Oral candidiasis is strongly associated with opportunist infection, and only a minority of patients presenting with KS alone will develop oral candidiasis.

The candidiasis of the mouth may be diagnosed clinically by the finding of plaques of 'thrush' on the buccal mucosa (Plate 5); these plaques are readily dislodged by a spatula, and may be taken for culture or wet slide microscopy for fungal hyphae. The plaques may be seen on all mucosal surfaces, but are particularly prominent on the underside of the tongue. In this site, candidiasis must be distinguished from leucoplakia (see above). The leucoplakia lesions are not dislodged on examination.

As throat swabs in healthy persons not infrequently grow *Candida* spp. as a normal oral flora, the diagnosis of oral candidiasis should be a clinical one, with microbiological confirmation, rather than vice versa. A positive culture for *Candida* from a throat swab is not evidence of oral candidiasis.

Candidal infection in AIDS may extend to the oesophagus, with plaques of *Candida* extending to the stomach. These may be asymptomatic, but usually cause an aching retrosternal discomfort on swallowing liquids or solids. Oesophageal candidiasis may be readily demonstrated by a barium swallow (see Plate 8), with glucagon or Buscopan to relax the oesophageal smooth musculature, or by oesophagoscopy. The significance of candidal overgrowth through the length of the bowel has yet to be established. It is possible that candidal infection of the jejunum is responsible for some of the malabsorption syndrome seen in AIDS.

Oral candidiasis may be treated with local treatment (e.g. nystatin suspension, Fungilin lozenges, etc.) but is not always controlled by these topical measures, and may necessitate the use of systemic treatment with ketoconazole (200 mg OD/BD). Oesophageal candidiasis is an indication for long-term ketoconazole, in an attempt to avoid dissemination of candidal infection. The recently reported hepatotoxicity of ketoconazole does not appear to be any more common in the context of HTLV-III infection, and this drug should continue to be used for the management of candidiasis in AIDS.

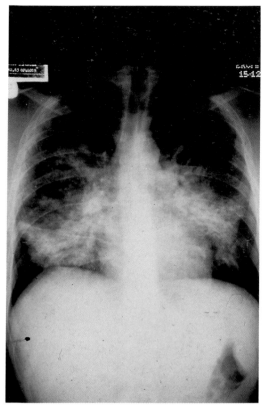

Plate 1. Chest X-ray, showing *Pneumocystis carinii* pneumonia

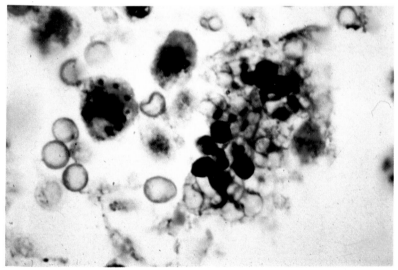

Plate 2. Transbronchial biopsy with silver stain, showing cysts of *Pneumocystis carinii*

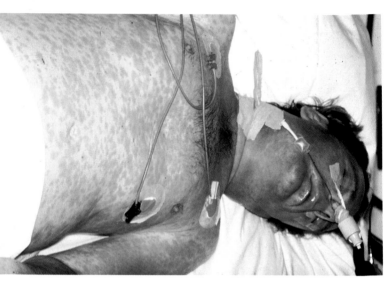

Plate 3. Maculopapular skin rash to co-trimoxazole in context of AIDS, in patient with no prior sulphonamide allergy

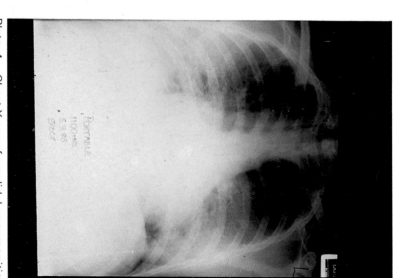

Plate 4. Chest X-ray of candidal pneumonitis in AIDS

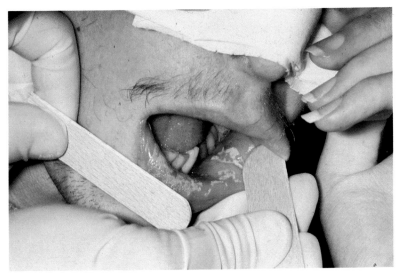

Plate 5. Plaques of oral candidiasis

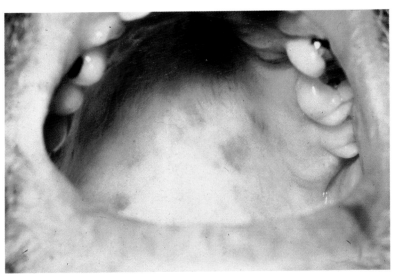

Plate 6. Oral lesions of Kaposi's sarcoma on hard and soft palate

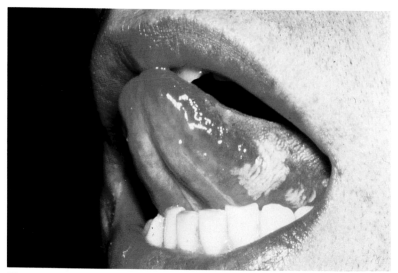

Plate 7.   Oral hairy leucoplakia on lateral border of tongue, in man with PGL

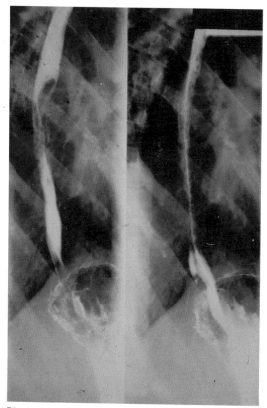

Plate 8.   Barium swallow, showing plaques of oesophageal candidiasis

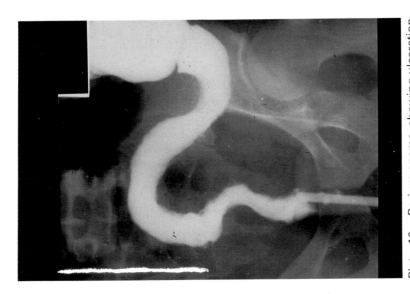

Plate 10. Barium enema, showing ulceration of rectum and sigmoid colon due to infiltration by Kaposi's sarcoma

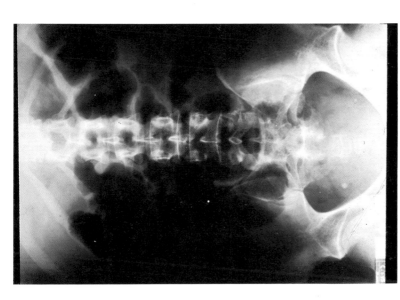

Plate 9. Plain abdominal X-ray, showing generalised large bowel distension due to CMV colitis

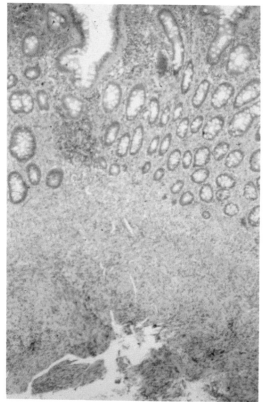

Plate 11. Rectal biopsy, showing KS infiltration in smooth muscle layer, with
superficial chronic inflammatory
changes (low-power)

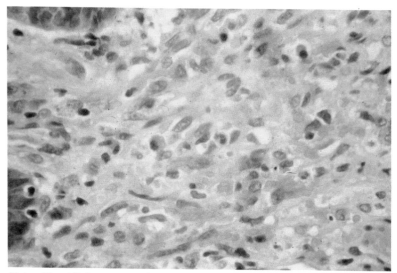

Plate 12. High-power micrograph of rectal biopsy, showing typical
features of KS, with extravasated red blood cells, spindle
cells and intracellular clefts

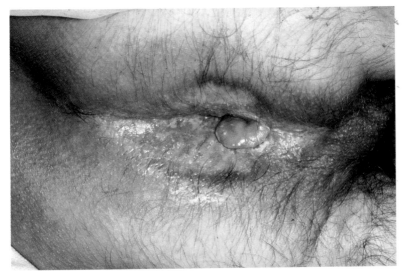

Plate 13. Peri-anal ulceration due to herpes simplex, in context of AIDS

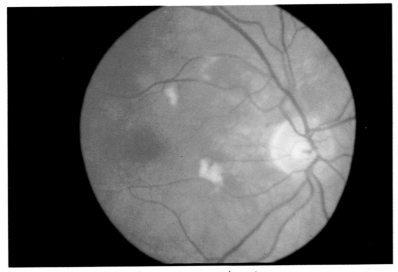

Plate 14. Retina with three cotton-wool spots

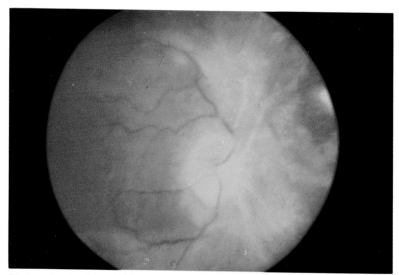

Plate 15. CMV retinitis

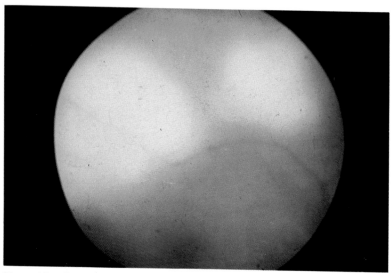

Plate 16. Probable candidal infection of retina and posterior chamber

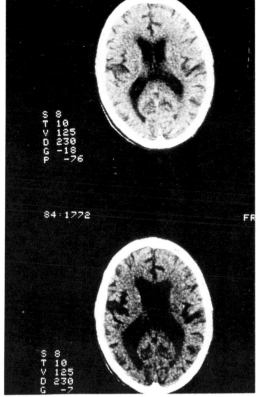

Plate 17. Unenhanced CT scan of brain, showing progressive cerebral atrophy associated with AIDS encephalopathy; two cuts taken 9 months apart

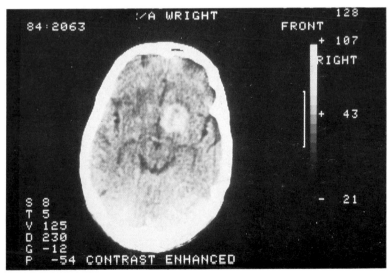

Plate 18. Enhanced CT scan in patient with hemiparesis, showing enhancing lesion of right parietal lobe, due to *Toxoplasma* brain abscess, with low-density non-enhancing lesion in left parietal lobe

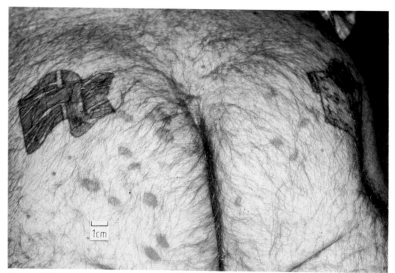

Plate 19.   Lesions of KS on buttocks

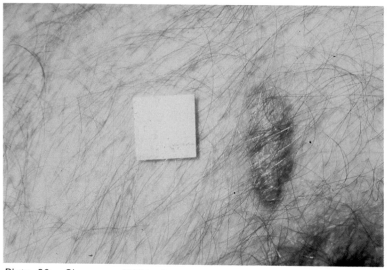

Plate 20.   Close-up of KS lesion

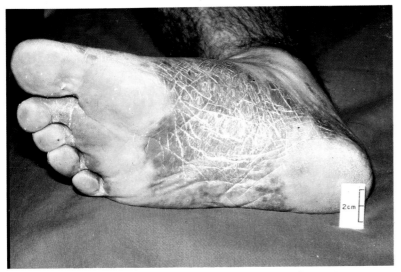

Plate 21. Hyperpigmentation of KS lesion after interferon therapy

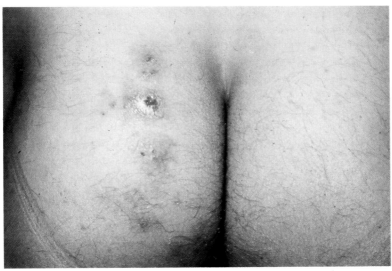

Plate 22. Persistent herpes simplex infection on buttock in patient with PGL

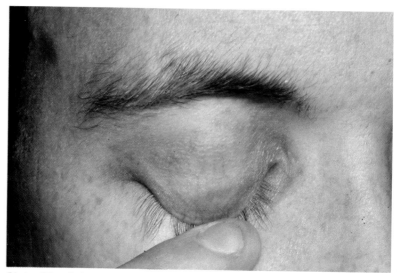

Plate 23. Seborrhoeic eczema on eyelid in patient with AIDS

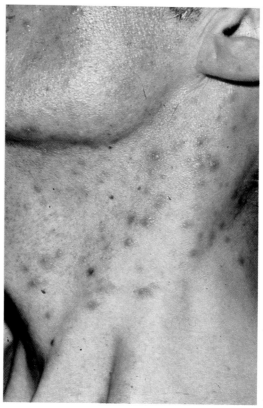

Plate 24. Facial folliculitis in patient with PGL

Cryptosporidiosis   The protozoan parasite *Cryptosporidium* has been known to be a cause of diarrhoea in cattle, but has only recently emerged as a serious pathogen in man. In AIDS the symptoms are of a persistent high-volume diarrhoea with large quantities of watery stool. This diarrhoea has been shown to be secretory in origin, although the mechanism is unclear. The diagnosis is made by the staining of stool (unconcentrated is normally sufficient) with an acid–alcohol-fast stain by which the cryptosporidial oocysts stain acid-fast.

The diarrhoea of this infection is not treatable with conventional anti-diarrhoeal agents, and as yet it is not possible to eradicate the parasite. In AIDS this infection has been fatal in the majority of cases, with symptoms persisting over a period of months. Therapy is limited to supportive measures and replacement of fluid and electrolytes. Although early reports of the use of spiramycin were enthusiastic, it now appears that this drug will not eradicate the organism. An effective treatment for this devastating infection is urgently required.

Salmonella, Shigella and Other Enterobacteria   While still omitted from the CDC definition of AIDS, infection with *Salmonella typhimurium* has presented a considerable clinical problem in AIDS in the UK and elsewhere. This bacterium is a facultative intracellular pathogen, and therefore requires a functioning cellular immune system for its elimination. In AIDS small infecting doses, as may be found in battery-raised poultry, produce an enteritis followed by a bacteraemia which may be persistent and unresponsive to appropriate chemotherapy. While the *Salmonella* enteritis is manageable, and the symptoms are not necessarily severe, the bacteraemia and its consequences of fever and tissue invasion may be debilitating.

The danger of AIDS patients acquiring *Salmonella* or *Shigella* infection, and then developing a persistent bacteraemia, is a reason to recommend caution in exposure to poorly cooked poultry in these patients.

Although *Giardia lamblia* and *Entamoeba histolytica* are common infections in homosexual men, these organisms pose no special risk to the patient with AIDS, who deals with these pathogens in an apparently normal manner.

Herpes Virus Family   After oral candidiasis, infection of the peri-anal region with herpes simplex type 2 virus (HSV) is the commonest infection of the gut in homosexual patients with AIDS. This infection produces florid, persisting ulcerating lesions, which may resemble piles clinically by the swelling and oedema surrounding the deep ulcers at the anal margin (see Plate 13). There may be bleeding on defaecation, and tenesmus, but peri-anal HSV infection is not a cause of diarrhoea. The infection can extend into the anal canal and into the rectum itself. The lesions may reach a considerable size and spread to the buttocks, and do not resemble the classical vesicular genital HSV.

Any ulcerating lesion of the peri-anal region must be examined carefully and cultured for herpes simplex, and a diagnosis of syphilis excluded by dark-ground microscopy or serology. Lesions on the anal margin which are culture-negative for HSV, and which have failed to respond to acyclovir, should be biopsied, to exclude squamous carcinoma.

Peri-oral herpes simplex is seen in AIDS patients, as a chronic, low-grade persistent infection, but without the severe ulceration seen in the peri-anal area. Management with prophylactic acyclovir is effective, and the daily dose of acyclovir may be reduced as far as possible; some patients are controlled on as little as 200 mg/day.

Cytomegalovirus (CMV) Infection   CMV may invade the large bowel in patients with AIDS, to produce CMV colitis. This condition presents with recurrent bouts of continuous watery diarrhoea, with the passage of blood with the stool, abdominal pain and distension, occasionally with marked rebound tenderness, and fever. Plain abdominal X-rays during a bout of distension show gross dilatation of the large bowel, sometimes with scanty fluid levels (see Plate 9). Diagnosis may be made by histological examination of a rectal or colonoscopic biopsy, showing invasive CMV with typical inclusions within the smooth muscle layer; CMV viral culture may be positive in the stool, urine and blood during the acute attacks. In patients with more continuous infection, chronic diarrhoea and loss of weight will occur, with a persistent low-grade fever.

CMV may also affect the upper bowel to produce oesophageal ulceration. These ulcers may be large (up to 5 cm), and cause considerable dysphagia; as with CMV colitis, fever is a common sign, and the diagnosis may be confirmed at biopsy.

Treatment of invasive CMV infection has previously been extremely poor. However, the emergence of foscarnet (Phosphonoformate, Astra Pharmaceuticals), and latterly DHPG, an analogue of acyclovir, is enabling active therapy of CMV infection to be undertaken.

Kaposi's Sarcoma of the Gut   Although KS is primarily recognised as a skin tumour, it is a multifocal tumour of endothelial origin that may affect virtually any site, but seems to have a predilection for the gastro-intestinal system. Any part of the gut may be affected, from mouth to anus. GI lesions are almost invariably associated with lesions of KS on the hard or soft palate, and these oral lesions should always be sought (see Plate 6).

Most of the GI KS lesions are silent, often found as nodules on the mucosal wall, or plaques of KS without ulceration. Some patients will develop significant infiltration of the gut, leading to colicky abdominal pains, ulceration of the mucosa with bleeding, and stricture of the bowel; in severe cases this may resemble ulcerative colitis clinically (see barium enema, Plate 10). The histology of ulcerating lesions of the gut secondary to infiltration by KS shows that the tumour lies deep to the submucosa, within the muscle layer. Therefore, a deep rectal biopsy is required, as superficial biopsies may show chronic inflammatory changes only, adding to the confusion with inflammatory bowel disorders (see Plates 11 and 12). The treatment of gastro-intestinal KS is discussed on page 28.

Table 1.11 Treatment of GI infection in AIDS

Organism	Diagnosis	Treatment	Adverse effects
Cryptosporidium	Stool ZN stain Biopsy	Supportive	
Candida spp.	Culture Barium swallow Oesophagoscopy	Fungilin lozenges Nystatin suspension Ketoconazole, 200 mg/d	 Rash Hepatotoxic ? Adrenal suppression
Herpes simplex	Culture EM	Acyclovir, 200 mg 5 × /d Maintain 200 mg/d	 Rash
CMV	Culture Biopsy	Foscarnet, i.v. 0.08 mg kg^{-1} min^{-1} DHPG, i.v.	Bone deposition ?
Salmonella	Culture blood/ stool	Check antibiotic sensitivities Chloramphenicol Ampicillin Mecillinam etc.	

Central Nervous System (CNS) Presentation

The CNS is the third major organ system to be infected by opportunist pathogens or tumours in AIDS. The commonest infection is cryptococcal meningitis, a fungal meningitis which frequently presents not with photophobia and neck stiffness, but with fever, variable headache, midline ataxia and mild disturbance of gait. Cryptococcal meningitis is commonly seen as part of the presentation of disseminated infection.

As with other infections in AIDS, the signs of CNS disease may be atypical. Toxoplasmosis in AIDS presents as an infection entirely localised to the CNS, causing intracerebral brain abscesses, frequently with long tract signs. The clinical picture of CNS disease is further complicated by the 'AIDS encephalopathy', a condition similar to presenile dementia which occurs in up to 40% of patients with established AIDS.

The clinical problems of the CNS may be divided into focal lesions, diffuse lesions and lesions of the retina (see Table 1.12).

Table 1.12 Clinical signs of CNS infection in AIDS

Symptoms	Headache
	Disturbance of gait or balance
	Disturbance of visual acuity
	Focal or general fits
	Disturbance of higher centres
Signs	Meningism
	Long tract signs (hemiparesis)
	Abnormal optic fundi
	Midline cerebellar signs (especially ataxia)
	Higher centres (memory, cerebration)
Organisms	*Cryptococcus* − meningitis
	Toxoplasma − focal lesion, retinitis
	Candida − focal lesion
	Lymphoma − focal lesion
	Cytomegalovirus − retinitis, ? encephalitis
	Polyoma virus (JC/BK) − PML

Focal Lesions

Mass lesions on CT scan, frequently visualised with ring enhancement due to surrounding cerebral oedema or encephalitis, are a common presentation in AIDS, and are usually caused by *Toxoplasma gondii* brain abscess (see Plate 18). These abscesses may be multiple, and present with long tract pyramidal signs, or with focal or grand mal epilepsy. Areas of low density (encephalitis) may also be seen without enhancement. The *Toxoplasma* lesions are not necessarily associated with concurrent *Toxoplasma* retinitis. The differential diagnosis of a mass lesion in the CNS is primary B cell lymphoma, and candidal abscess. Both of these have been rare in the UK to date.

The diagnosis of CNS toxoplasmosis cannot reliably be made on the basis of positive *Toxoplasma* serology, either in serum or in CSF. A proportion of patients with negative serology at both sites will have proven CNS toxoplasmosis at post-mortem. However, a high titre for *Toxoplasma* in the context of a mass lesion in the brain will define a large proportion of patients. Rising titres may not be seen, owing to the polyclonal B cell activation seen in AIDS. Brain biopsy is the only reliable method of diagnosis, but this may be relatively contraindicated in the light of reports of increased morbidity and mortality following brain biopsy in AIDS. A high degree of clinical suspicion is warranted, and trial of anti-*Toxoplasma* treatment may be the most reliable method of diagnosis of a mass CNS lesion, with brain biopsy reserved for those patients who fail to respond to therapy, or whose presentations are atypical.

Treatment of CNS toxoplasmosis is by Fansidar (pyrimethamine/sulpha-doxine), initially 2 tablets BD for 3 weeks, followed by a reducing dosage to a maintenance of 1 tablet/week for life (see Table 1.13). The chance of relapse is high.

Table 1.13   Treatment of CNS infection in AIDS

Organism	Diagnosis	Treatment	Adverse effects
Cryptococcus	CSF: Gram India ink antigen Serum antigen Post Rx LP	Amphotericin* 5-Fluorocytosine ? 5 FC prophylaxis	See above
Toxoplasma	CT scan abscess Ring enhancing Serum antibody CSF antibody ? Biopsy	Fansidar 2 tab/BD (pyrimethamine/ sulphadoxine) Maintenance dose Add folinic acid	Bone marrow depression Rash
Candida	CT scan abscess Disseminated infection	Amphotericin* 5-Fluorocytosine	See above
CMV retinitis	Clinical appearance	DHPG ? Foscarnet	Not known
AIDS encephalopathy	Dementia CT scan atrophy	Supportive Control epilepsy	

*See Table 1.9 for dosage.

Diffuse Lesions

Fungal meningitis caused by *Cryptococcus neoformans* is the commonest infection in the cerebrospinal fluid (CSF), and usually presents with a midline ataxia, mild to severe frontal headaches, and fever. There may be subtle changes of higher cerebral function, with decreased concentration and difficulty with reading. There are, in general, no signs of classical meningism. The signs of ataxia may be minimal, with slight unsteadiness of gait, or a poor heel–toe walking test. Any patient with persistent headache alone, in the context of AIDS, should have a CSF examination with India ink or cryptococcal antigen study and fungal culture to exclude this organism. Our experience shows that patients have a prompt response to amphotericin and 5-fluorocytosine, and that recurrence is a relatively late event (up to 10 months). The role of anticryptococcal prophyl-axis or the monitoring of serum cryptococcal antigen is not yet established.

After treatment, a repeat lumbar puncture should be performed to establish elimination of the organism.

It would appear that herpes simplex and CMV encephalitis do occur in AIDS, but only rarely. CMV infection of the brain has been seen as a subacute encephalitis without localising signs, and as an apparent vasculitis, causing internuclear ophthalmoplegia and brain-stem lesions. Further natural history of CMV disease in the CNS will undoubtedly reveal further syndromes in the future.

The AIDS Encephalopathy

In 1982 Mildvan in New York noted that patients with established AIDS were developing a dementing illness, with a variable onset of change of personality, loss of short- and long-term memory and inability to cerebrate. Latterly, patients have presented prior to opportunist infection or tumour with a history of inability to function at work, and with alterations of personality. CT scanning of the brain reveals a marked atrophy of both white and grey matter, with dilatation of the ventricles (see Plate 17). This atrophy is progressive and may cause grand mal epilepsy in addition to dementia. This condition, termed the AIDS encephalopathy, is unrelated to any discernible opportunist infection, and post-mortem histology shows microglial nodules and neuronal loss only. Recently, Shaw has demonstrated that HTLV-III RNA and DNA are detectable in brain cells in this syndrome. This encephalopathy may therefore represent primary AIDS virus infection of the CNS.

Opportunist infections of the CNS may occasionally present with an encephalopathy, particularly cryptococcal meningitis and CMV encephalitis. As these infections may be treatable, the CSF must be examined before a diagnosis of AIDS encephalopathy is made.

There is no effective treatment for this condition at present, which affects as many as 40% of patients with AIDS. It is not known whether asymptomatic HTLV-III-infected patients will develop evidence of this encephalopathy over a prolonged time.

Retinal Lesions

The retina is a highly accessible organ for examination, and lesions of the optic fundi are of great clinical importance in AIDS. The commonest lesion is the 'cotton-wool spot', a soft exudate which arises suddenly, lasts approximately 6 weeks and may be seen in any part of the retina (see Plate 14). These lesions may occur in any patient with AIDS, and may arise prior to overt infection or tumour. Cotton-wool spots rarely interfere with visual acuity, and are benign; the pathogenesis of these lesions is unknown, but they resemble those seen in patients with vasculitis.

Diminution of visual acuity in patients with AIDS is an indication for urgent ophthalmological assessment. The most frequent cause is CMV retinitis; this is often a CMV-mediated arteritis of the retinal vasculature, leading to destruction of arterioles and infarction of distal retinal tissue. The appearances on examination are distinctive, with early narrowing and irregularity of the lumen of the retinal vessels, followed by vascular occlusion and the appearance of exudates and haemorrhages preceding the final infarction of the affected area of retina (see Plate 15). Isolated peripheral lesions of choroidoretinitis are also seen due to CMV, but interfere less with vision.

CMV retinitis poses a serious threat of blindness, and may be bilateral. Treatment of CMV retinitis with DHPG, a drug related to acyclovir, has shown promising efficacy in early clinical trials.

Other opportunist infections of the retina are uncommon, but may produce disturbance of vision and florid retinal changes. Plate 16 shows a presumptive candidal infection of the retina, in a patient presenting with a cerebral abscess.

Skin Manifestations of AIDS

Skin lesions in AIDS may be divided into Kaposi's sarcoma (KS) and infections of the skin secondary to immunosuppression. KS accounts for 25% of all initial presentations with AIDS, and a further 10% of patients will develop KS after opportunist infections. The skin lesions secondary to AIDS are diverse, and as yet not fully documented (see Table 1.14).

Table 1.14   Skin lesions in AIDS

(1) Tumours	Kaposi's sarcoma	
	Squamous carcinoma (? AIDS-related)	
	Lymphoma with skin involvement	
(2) Infections		
Local	Viral	Herpes simplex
		Herpes zoster
		Molluscum contagiosum
	Fungal	Tinea
		Pityrosporum
Disseminated		Histoplasmosis
		Cryptococcosis
(3) Non-specific	Seborrhoeic eczema	
	Folliculitis	
	Vasculitis (leucoclastic)	
	Xeroderma	

Kaposi's Sarcoma

KS is the major tumour of AIDS, and although primarily a tumour of skin, in AIDS any internal organ except for the CNS may be involved. As seen above, the gastro-intestinal tract is a favoured site for disseminated KS.

KS is thought to be a tumour of endothelial cell origin, and is multifocal, rather than spreading through metastasis. The tumour is locally invasive, but effects through space occupation rather than invasion seem to predominate. Any part of the skin may be affected. The tumour presents as a purple-coloured lesion in the skin or subcutaneous tissue, firm to palpate, non-tender, non-pruritic and, in general, elevated above surrounding skin (see Plates 19 and 20). Lesions may develop from new to 1 cm in diameter in 7–10 days. Lesions are usually multiple, and seldom more than 5 cm in diameter, although lesions may coalesce in late disease. However, some lesions have presented as macular rather than nodular, and may be small. A high index of suspicion should be entertained for any suspicious pigmented lesion in a high-risk patient, to enable early biopsy to be performed to establish a diagnosis.

Diagnosis is by skin biopsy, and, even in early lesions, the appearance of spindle-shaped cells, intracellular clefts and extravasated red blood cells is pathognomic for KS (see histology, Plates 11 and 12). Early lesions may lack these diagnostic markers, and the histological assessment of the macular lesions of early KS may be difficult.

Table 1.15 Treatment of Kaposi's sarcoma

(1) Local skin lesions	Biopsy for diagnosis
	If solitary, observe progress only
	Excise individual lesions if accessible
	If symptomatic (local pressure effects, peri-anal lesions), local radiotherapy
(2) Disseminated skin lesions	Biopsy for diagnosis — observe
	If number of lesions increases or symptoms develop, consider alpha-interferon 20 MU/m² — and maintain
(3) Disseminated visceral lesions	Biopsy for diagnosis
	Consider: alpha-interferon radiotherapy
	Chemotherapy: vincristine/vinblastine VP-16

Prior to treatment, staging of the KS lesions should be attempted. This should begin with a thorough clinical examination, with documentation of the size and distribution of the skin lesions; if multiple, photography may assist in assessing later response to therapy. If lesions are present on the hard or soft palate, investigation of the GI tract should be undertaken by endoscopy (preferably) or by barium examination, in order to assess the degree of gut infiltration. Chest X-ray and lung function testing may be a simple, non-invasive way of excluding major pulmonary involvement by KS; FOB and biopsy may be necessary in other cases. However, invasive investigation of an asymptomatic patient with skin lesions only must be seen to be less than productive, and possibly not in the best interests of the patient.

The treatment of KS is currently unsatisfactory. First, the prognosis for KS in AIDS is considerably better than for patients with opportunist infection. The course of KS is directly related to the degree of immunosuppression of the patient at presentation. This may be roughly quantified by the total lymphocyte count; patients with KS and lymphocytes $> 1.5 \times 10^9/l$ have an 80% chance of surviving 2 years, against a 20% survival in patients presenting with total lymphocyte count $< 1.0 \times 10^9/l$. Patients with KS alone have a better 2 year survival than those with KS and opportunist infection, or opportunist infection alone.

Therefore, any therapy for KS in the context of AIDS must not hasten the development of infection, lest the prognosis be worsened. Any cytotoxic chemotherapy which has been successful in the context of classical KS must be viewed with suspicion in the context of AIDS, owing to the heightened risk of marrow suppression and, hence, opportunist infection.

The treatment of isolated KS lesions on the skin may be by local excision if symptomatic, or by local radiotherapy if in a surgically inaccessible area. In mild cases with minimal skin lesions and a normal lymphocyte count, the lesions may best be left alone, and followed closely. Disseminated disease, whether confined to the skin or extending to viscera, is still poorly treatable. The mainstay of therapy at this time is alpha-interferon, used in high dose (20 MU/m^2) intramuscularly daily for 3 months, with long-term maintenance, usually with three-weekly injections. Although initial response to this drug is moderate, with less than 40% responders (partial or complete), early and late relapse are commonly seen. The pronounced malaise and weight loss caused by this dose of alpha-interferon are major problems, and may be a limiting factor in the widespread use of this drug. After successful therapy with alpha-interferon KS lesions regress, leaving hyperpigmented areas of skin (see Plate 21).

The use of cytotoxic chemotherapy has been reported with some success, particularly therapy using drugs with minimal marrow depression. In one trial with vincristine, good efficacy against KS was seen, with little increase in incidence of opportunist infection. Volberding has reported the use of vinblastine to be effective, but there was a higher rate of progression to opportunist infection in the treated group. The use of VP-16 has shown similarly good response rates for KS, and with an acceptable incidence of infection. More potent drugs such as Adriamycin have led to unacceptable rates of infection. Trials of combination therapy with interferon and cytotoxic drugs are currently under way. However, alpha-interferon must be seen as the first line of approach for the treatment of AIDS (KS) at this time, pending the results of trials in progress.

Skin Infection

Table 1.14 shows the possible skin lesions of AIDS recognised to date; undoubtedly more manifestations will be seen. Of the infections, herpes simplex is predominantly peri-anal in distribution, and peri-oral HSV has been uncommon as a clinical problem; these lesions are discussed above.

Herpes (varicella) zoster is seen commonly in the prodromal illness, but is unusual in frank AIDS. The rash of molluscum contagiosum is commonly seen on the face, and while difficult to eradicate (liquid nitrogen or 5% phenol applied locally), it is not dangerous to the patient. The fungal infections may be florid, but respond to the normal antifungal topical applications. Diagnosis of these fungal skin lesions is best made by skin scrapings and culture.

The skin lesions of disseminated infection are all atypical, and diagnosis follows biopsy rather than clinical appearance. Fungaemia of all causes may result in skin lesions, particularly cryptococcosis and histoplasmosis. Any atypical skin lesion in an AIDS patient should be biopsied if the diagnosis is not clinically apparent.

The non-specific skin lesions of AIDS are predominantly seborrhoeic eczema and facial folliculitis. The eczema arises in patients with no prior history of skin disease, and may be florid, affecting the face with marked cracking in skin folds. Atopic eczema may recur in patients with a history of atopy, eczema or asthma in childhood. The eczema may be controlled with aqueous cream and low-dose hydrocortisone cream topically. The facial folliculitis usually responds to Quinaderm.

Lymphadenopathic Presentation of AIDS

A proportion of patients with AIDS will present with lymphadenopathy only, with lymph node infection by opportunist fungal or mycobacterial agent, or with infiltration by Kaposi's sarcoma or lymphoma. Lymphadenopathic KS may precede, or occur in the absence of, cutaneous KS. Castleman's syndrome, hypervascular hyperplastic lymphadenopathy, has also been observed in the context of AIDS, presenting with giant splenomegaly, pancytopenia, lymphadenopathy and hepatomegaly. In this condition the lymph nodes may show small areas of infiltration by KS, often around the capsular margin. More extensive development of KS may follow this presentation.

The lymphoma associated with AIDS has been rare in the UK. Ziegler has reported 90 cases of non-Hodgkin's lymphoma in homosexual men in the USA. The lymphomas were B cell in origin, and 62% were high-grade (aggressive), compared with only 7% with low-grade histology. All but two patients in this series had extranodal lymphoma, with the CNS, bone marrow, bowel and mucocutaneous sites being the most frequently affected. In half the patients presenting with lymphadenopathy, AIDS developed after the diagnosis of non-Hodgkin's lymphoma. The patients were treated with standard combination chemotherapy, or radiotherapy, or both, and mortality in all histological grades was higher than currently reported rates in other patient populations.

The differential diagnosis of lymphadenopathic AIDS presentations is given in Table 1.16; this may be compared with Table 1.2, describing the differential diagnosis of PGL.

Table 1.16 Lymphadenopathic presentation of AIDS

Cause	Features
Kaposi's sarcoma	May occur without skin disease LN biopsy may show small foci only
Lymphoma	Skin involvement occurs early CNS extension common Extranodal involvement usual
Castleman's syndrome	Splenomegaly/hepatomegaly Pancytopenia/thrombocytopenia May be associated with KS in LN
Infection	Mycobacterial Fungal (especially cryptococcal)

SUMMARY

Although the infections and tumours of AIDS may seem to be in profusion and confusion, the principles behind the disease are straightforward. Infections may be multiple in any one patient, but a knowledge of the possible range of the syndrome and the most common presentations will enable a logical clinical path to be followed through the affected organs.

BIBLIOGRAPHY

General Textbooks on STD

Holmes, K. and Mardh, P. A. (1984). In Sparling, P. F. and Wiesner, P. J. (Eds.), *Sexually Transmitted Diseases*. New York, McGraw-Hill

King, Nichol and Roden (Eds.) (1980). *Venereal Diseases*, 4th Edn. London. Baillière Tindall

Ma, P. and Armstrong, D. (1984). *AIDS and Infections of Homosexual Men*. New York, Yorke Medical Books

Reviews on AIDS

AIDS (1983). UCLA Conference. Moderator: Gottlieb, M. S. *Ann. Int. Med.*, **99**, 208

AIDS – Clinical, Epidemiologic, Immunologic and Therapeutic Considerations (1984). NIH Conference. Moderator: Fauci, A. S. *Ann. Int. Med.*, **100**, 92

Harris, J. R. W. and Weber, J. N. (1984). AIDS. In Ferguson, A. (Ed.), *Advanced Medicine*, Vol. 20. London, Pitman

Pinching, A. J. (1984). AIDS. *Hospital Update*, 117

AIDS – An update (1985). NIH Conference. Moderator: Fauci, A. S. *Ann. Int. Med.*, **102**, 800

Epidemiology

Members of the Task Force on AIDS, CDC, Atlanta (1983). National case control study of Kaposi's sarcoma and *Pneumocystis carinii* pneumonia in homosexual men: Part 1, Epidemiologic results; Part 2, Laboratory results. *Ann. Int. Med.*, **99**, 145

Centres for Disease Control (1984). Update: AIDS – United States. *MMWR*, **33**, 661

Centres for Disease Control (1985). Update: AIDS – Europe. *MMWR*, **34**, 21

PGL

Mathur-Wagh, U., Enlow, R. W., Spigland, I. *et al.* (1984). Longitudinal study of PGL in homosexual men: Relation to AIDS. *Lancet*, **i**, 1033

Abrams, D. I., Lewis, B. J., Beckstead, J. H. *et al.* (1984). Persistent diffuse lymphadenopathy in homosexual men: endpoint or prodrome? *Ann. Int. Med.*, **100**, 801

Walsh, C. M., Nardi, M. A. and Karpatkin, S. (1984). On the mechanism of thrombocytopenic purpura in homosexual men. *New Engl. J. Med.*, **311**, 635

Greenspan, D., Greenspan, J., Conant, M. *et al.* (1984). Oral hairy leucoplakia in male homosexuals: evidence of association with both papilloma virus and a herpes-group virus. *Lancet*, **ii**, 831

Infections in AIDS

Cooper, D. A., Gold, J., MacLean, P. *et al.* (1985). Acute AIDS retrovirus infection. *Lancet*, **i**, 537

Engelberg, L. A., Lerner, C. W. and Tapper, M. L. (1984). Clinical features of *Pneumocystis carinii* pneumonia in AIDS. *Am. Rev. Respir. Dis.*, **130**, 689

Stover, D. E., White, D. A., Romano, P. A. *et al.* (1985). Spectrum of pulmonary disease associated with AIDS. *Am. J. Med.*, **78**, 429

Butkus Small, C., Harris, C. A., Friedland, G. H. and Klein, R. S. (1985). Treatment of PCP in AIDS. *Arch. Intern. Med.*, **145**, 837

Jacobs, J. L., Gold, J. W., Murray, H. W. *et al.* (1985). Salmonella infections in patients with AIDS. *Ann. Int. Med.*, **102**, 186

Kotler, D. P., Gaetz, H. P., Lange, M. *et al.* (1984). Enteropathy associated with AIDS. *Ann. Int. Med.*, **101**, 421

Snider, W. D., Simpson, D. M., Nielsen, S. *et al.* (1983). Neurological complications of AIDS: Analysis of 50 patients. *Ann. Neurol.*, **14**, 403

Shaw, G. M., Harper, M. E., Hahn, B. H. *et al.* (1985). HTLV-III infection in brains of children and adults with AIDS encephalopathy. *Science, N.Y.*, **227**, 177

Groopman, J. E., Gottlieb, M. S., Goodman, J. *et al.* (1984). Recombinant alpha-2 interferon therapy for Kaposi's sarcoma associated with AIDS. *Ann. Int. Med.*, **100**, 671

Ziegler, J. L., Beckstaed, J. A., Volberding, P. A. *et al.* (1984). Non-Hodgkins lymphoma in 90 homosexual men. *New Engl. J. Med.*, **311**, 565

2

Immunology: Immunological Profile, Pathogenesis and the Role of Diagnostic Tests

Anthony Pinching

INTRODUCTION

Until the AIDS epidemic, knowledge about cellular immune mechanisms among practising clinicians and health care workers was sketchy; opportunist infections in the immunocompromised host were regarded as recherché and as lists of bizarre organisms to be taken out and dusted down at rare intervals with a sense of the exotic; most lay people had no idea what immunologists were, unless something to do with vaccination; clinicians regarded them as laboratory-based scientists whose language was opaque, whose concepts were rarefied and whose relevance was doubtful; immunologists had uncertainties about the nature of immunosuppression in different contexts and were still grappling with the relevance of immunological tests, both new and old, to clinical diagnosis. AIDS has changed all that.

As a result of this tragic disease, we have learnt about the clinical effects of profound cellular immune deficiency, the widening spectrum of human retroviral disease, the basic mechanisms underlying immune competence and the effector cells concerned; we have been reminded about the potentially biohazardous nature of all patients and the need to apply common-sense and good technique to all those we care for, whether on the wards, in the laboratories or in the community; we have learnt about many areas of human society, from detailed aspects of life-style among high-risk groups to the behaviour of the press and those who administer the health service; perhaps most importantly, we have learnt about ourselves and our attitudes. While no one would have wished to see such a disease, it must be some small comfort to those affected by it that it has probably done more than any other single disease to teach us about science, medicine and society; but if AIDS has been a learning experience, it has also been a chastening and a humbling one.

  This chapter will attempt to outline our current view of AIDS as an immuno-deficiency disease, which was, after all, how it was first recognised and how it got its name; while we now also perceive it as part of the spectrum of an infectious disease, it is still crucial to examine it biologically and diagnostically from an immunological perspective. Some of the clinical features that tell us about its immunological nature will be re-emphasised, on the principle that most of what we know and need to know about the disease will be 'told' us by the patients, if we listen carefully. After a brief 'revision course' on the immune system, the immunological profile of AIDS is outlined as a background to an analysis of pathogenetic mechanisms; the immunological changes seen in other manifestations of HTLV-III infection are then discussed in the context of changes seen in other viral infections; and the relevance of diagnostic tests is put into perspective. Finally, approaches to treatment and prevention based on our current understanding of the disease are considered.

CLINICAL EVIDENCE FOR IMMUNODEFICIENCY

The Clinical Pattern

The cellular immune deficiency that characterises AIDS is the susceptibility to a special group of opportunist infections or virus-associated tumours, which we shall term 'opportunist tumours'. These secondary conditions determine the protean clinical manifestations of AIDS. The major infections, which are desscribed in detail in Chapter 1, comprise *Pneumocystis carinii* pneumonia, disseminated cytomegalovirus (CMV) infection, herpes simplex ulceration, mucosal candidiasis, cerebral toxoplasmosis, disseminated mycobacterial infections (atypical or tuberculosis), cryptococcosis, salmonellosis and cryptosporidiosis. Such a pattern of infections is reminiscent of that seen in patients with cellular immune deficiency; for example, in children with severe combined immune deficiency or in patients receiving high-dose steroids for organ transplantation or systemic lupus erythematosus (SLE).

Opportunist Infections

What is meant by the term 'opportunist infection'? Opportunist micro-organisms are those that take advantage of a defect in host defence to give rise to disease that they would not normally cause. They include the following: (1) Those that do not normally cause any disease in the normal host (e.g. *Pneumocystis*, atypical mycobacteria). (2) Those that can affect the normal host but causing disease which is mild, localised and self-limiting (e.g. oral or genital herpes simplex, mononucleosis due to *Toxoplasma* or CMV, or transient enteritis due to *Cryptosporidium*). In the compromised patient the pattern of disease is distinctive, being severe, disseminated and persistent: herpes causes progressive ulceration;

Toxoplasma causes cerebral abscesses or encephalitis; CMV may disseminate variously as pneumonitis, oesophageal ulceration, enteritis, colitis, adrenalitis, retinitis or a subacute encephalitis; and cryptosporidial gut infection causes persistent torrential cholera-like diarrhoea with malabsorption. (3) Those that are conventional pathogens (e.g. *Mycobacterium tuberculosis*), which in AIDS patients leads to disseminated disease that may respond poorly to antituberculous therapy.

Opportunist Tumours

The common opportunist tumours seen are: (1) Kaposi's sarcoma and (2) B cell lymphoma. These may present in unusual forms and are apparently multifocal: Kaposi's sarcoma has an atypical cutaneous distribution and, in some patients, shows visceral, especially gastro-intestinal or lymph node, involvement; the B cell lymphomas, usually Burkitt-like non-Hodgkin's lymphoma, have a high frequency of extranodal involvement. This pattern of tumours is broadly familiar from patients on long-term immunosuppressive therapy. There is suggestive evidence that these tumours arise in the immunocompromised host as a result of oncogenesis by human herpesviruses: CMV for Kaposi's sarcoma and Epstein-Barr virus (EBV) for the B cell lymphomas.

Differences Between AIDS and Other Cellular Immunodeficiencies

When contrasted with other patients with compromised cellular immunity, it is evident that, for AIDS patients, 'the rules are different'. The difference results from the more profound defect in host defence, clinical evidence of the secondary manifestations being blunted and more insidious. The failure of host response results in less tissue infiltration, including failure to make granulomas and unreliable serological responses. Thus, *Pneumocystis* infections may develop insidiously over weeks or months, in contrast to the rapid progression over a few days seen in transplant patients. Mycobacterial disease, especially with atypical organisms, resembles lepromatous leprosy, with numerous organisms but negligible evidence of host response. CMV causes more disseminated disease than has been seen hitherto, with novel complications such as oesophageal ulcers, malabsorption, colitis and adrenal insufficiency. Serological responses to CMV and *Toxoplasma* are unreliable diagnostically, either because antibody titres are non-specifically raised and show no further rise during reactivation or because a primary antibody response may be absent.

Infection at Different Stages of the Immunodeficiency

Organisms of high virulence, such as *Mycobacterium tuberculosis*, can give rise to infection when immunodeficiency is slight and so tend to occur relatively early in the course of AIDS. Similarly, the emergence of Kaposi's sarcoma alone, especially in the limited cutaneous form, reflects relatively less severe immuno-deficiency. By contrast, disseminated infection with low-grade pathogens such as atypical mycobacteria occur relatively late in the course. CMV-induced disease appears to occur relatively late and is associated with poor prognosis; this may be because it only occurs when immunodeficiency is severe, or because its own immunosuppressive effects are added to those of HTLV-III, compounding the cellular defect.

Other Determinants of the Pattern of Infection

The infective and malignant complications of AIDS also reflect the organisms latent in or carried by the host. These will in turn be determined by where a person has been and what he has done. In this way, AIDS patients project their previous microbial exposure onto the secondary disease they develop when their cellular immunity becomes critically impaired. This accounts for variations in opportunist infections seen in AIDS patients from different life-styles and geo-graphical areas. These include: a high prevalence of *Salmonella* infection in the UK and Europe; the different patterns of atypical mycobacteria in the UK (*Mycobacterium xenopii* and *M. kansasii*) and in the USA (*M. avium-intracellu-lare*); the occurrence of *M. tuberculosis* infection in populations with high latency; histoplasmosis and strongyloidiasis in patients who have resided in endemic areas, often many years before; and the high frequency of CMV infec-tions among homosexual men, in whom CMV may be sexually transmitted (the latter fact may also account for the high frequency of Kaposi's sarcoma in this group compared with other groups).

AN OUTLINE OF THE IMMUNE SYSTEM

General Organisation

Before the immunological features of AIDS are considered, an outline of the immune system is provided, including a scheme for the functional interactions between its constituent cells. There are a number of effectors which may be specific (antibody, cytotoxic T cells) or non-specific (complement, neutrophils, eosinophils, monocytes, macrophages, natural killer and killer lymphocytes). Their activity is regulated by T helper cells and T suppressor cells, while the induction of the immune response is determined by the presentation of specific antigens to lymphocytes on specialised antigen-presenting cells (macrophages, Langerhans cells and dendritic cells).

Antibodies and Antibody-dependent Phagocytic Effector Cells

Antibodies are produced following maturation of B cells into plasma cells. Antigen-specific B cells proliferate on exposure to antigen, which is usually 'seen' on antigen-presenting cells. These B cells then undergo differentiation and clonal expansion into antibody-secreting plasma cells, under the control of humoral factors. Antibodies provide an antigen-specific system which may act alone in host defence-specific humoral immunity; however, they also provide a system of recognition for non-specific effectors – complement, phagocytes and killer cells. For phagocytes (neutrophils, eosinophils, monocytes and tissue macrophages), this function is termed opsonisation, and is concerned with ingestion, killing and/or digestion of microbial organisms. Thus, non-specific effectors are provided with specificity by antibody; antigen recognition is achieved by the Fab portion of antibody, while its Fc portion is detected by Fc receptors on the cells. Complement C3b, generated following activation of classical or alternative pathways, provides an additional non-specific system for the recognition of micro-organisms by cells. Opsonisation efficiency is greatly enhanced by interaction of C3b with C3b receptors, and triggering of C3b receptors also promotes optimal intracellular killing.

Three Types of Lymphocyte with Cytotoxic Function

For *killer lymphocytes*, antibody-dependent cellular cytotoxicity (ADCC) is typically directed against host cells that have been altered antigenically by viral infection. Again specificity is conferred on non-specific effectors by antibody. *Natural killer cells*, which are of uncertain lineage but are probably T-cell-related, are non-specific effectors that are able to kill some virally infected and tumour cells. They have been loosely associated with phenotypic markers, Leu7 and, more specifically, Leu11. Killer and natural killer populations probably overlap. This may be in the same sense that phagocytes can ingest and kill organisms without antibody, but do so more efficiently and for a wider range of targets with antibody. Among the most important cellular effectors are the *cytotoxic T cells*, which show antigen-specific cytotoxicity and are important for elimination of virus-infected cells.

T Cells and Macrophage Activation

Other antigen-specific T cells, termed delayed-type hypersensitivity (DTH) T cells, collaborate with macrophages in the mediation of DTH responses, largely through release of macrophage-activating lymphokines, including gamma-interferon. This mechanism of macrophage activation is crucial to the elimination of the facultative intracellular pathogens (e.g. *Listeria, Toxoplasma, Salmonella*, and various fungi and mycobacteria). It may also be important in the killing of *Pneumocystis carinii* and in the elimination of herpes viruses. This is another example where specific mechanisms have conferred specificity upon non-specific effectors – in this instance, macrophages.

Humoral Regulators of Cellular Immunity

The proliferation of T cells is, like that of B cells, dependent on lymphokines and monokines, the humoral mediators of cellular immune responsiveness. Interleukin 1 (IL-1) is released from macrophages and serves to trigger T cells to produce interleukin 2 (IL-2 or T cell growth factor). IL-2 not only stimulates the growth of T cells directly, but also amplifies its action by increasing their expression of IL-2 receptors. Gamma-interferon and other lymphokines are also produced by activated T helper/DTH cells and lead to activation of macrophages; this greatly enhances their capacity to kill intracellular pathogens. In addition, all the interferons, gamma- (immune), beta- (fibroblast) and alpha- (leucocyte), are able to stimulate the production and the functional activity of natural killer cells.

Cellular Regulation and the Induction of the Immune Response

The production and/or activity of these various effector cells is controlled by regulatory T cells, termed helper and suppressor T cells. These may either act directly on effectors or on one another. Induction of the immune response, whether humoral (B cell) or cellular (T cell), results from the interaction between antigen, generally as presented on antigen-presenting cells in the context of self- (HLA) and antigen-specific T cells, whether inducers or suppressors. Immuno-genetic diversity is seen in the HLA (tissue type) antigens, which in part determine differing immune responsiveness among different members of a population. Antigen recognition is achieved by specificities in the antibody or T cell receptor repertoire, generated by gene rearrangements in B and T cell populations; the two systems of recognition appear to respond to different antigenic determinants (epitopes).

Cellular Communication in the Immune System

The immune system comprises mobile single cells that act in co-operation with other cells or on cellular targets. Unlike the cells of the nervous system, they are not permanently connected to the cells with which they interact; they therefore require a system of communication to enable function. The expression of HLA antigens provides a part of this recognition system. Cells bearing HLA Class I antigens (A, B and C) are recognised by a subset of T cells bearing the differentiation antigen T8, while those bearing the Class II HLA (D, DR) antigens are recognised by T cells bearing the T4 antigen. These phenotypic markers T4 and T8 are identified by monoclonal antibodies. In this way the complementary recognition molecules, T4-Class II and T8-Class I, provide the basic language of the immune system.

Relationship between Phenotype and Function

When first identified, it was thought that T4 and T8 were markers for function, because T4 cells showed predominantly helper or inducer functions *in vitro*, while T8 cells showed mainly suppressor or cytotoxic functions. T4 cells also appeared to be the lymphocyte type involved in DTH responses. However, the phenotypes are only broadly related to function: for example, T4 cells may be cytotoxic (for cells bearing Class II antigens) and are necessary for suppressor function to be expressed by T8 cells. Despite the current perception that lymphocyte phenotypes reflect the language of the immune system, they are still frequently referred to as 'helper' (T4) and 'suppressor' (T8) lymphocytes.

Other phenotypic markers have now been identified which further subdivide these sub-populations and appear again to enrich for certain functions. T4 cells may be divided according to whether or not they express Leu8; the sub-set bearing T4 and not Leu8 mainly provide help for immunoglobulin production, while the complementary T4+, Leu8+ population are mainly involved in inducer and/or DTH function. Again, these markers may reflect recognition signals rather than functional activity.

THE IMMUNOLOGICAL FEATURES OF AIDS

T Lymphocytes

The best evidence for the type of immunodeficiency in AIDS is the pattern of opportunist disease seen clinically. Man in his environment is the ultimate bioassay for the function of the immune system. However, the characteristic immunological profile in laboratory studies confirms that the primary defect is one of cellular immunity. This profile has also provided the means for dissecting pathogenetic mechanisms. Its role in diagnosis will be discussed later. Patients are typically lymphopenic, and this is due to a reduction in the number of circulating T cells. It is specifically the T4 'helper/inducer' phenotype that is depleted; the complementary T8 'suppressor/cytotoxic' phenotype is unaffected. The reduction in circulating T4 cells appears to reflect a reduction in tissue T4 cells. Furthermore, it appears to be the Leu8+ sub-set of T4 cells that is lost in AIDS patients — i.e. cells that are least involved in help for immunoglobulin production and more concerned with inducer and delayed-type hypersensitivity function.

Many AIDS patients have significant numbers of T4 cells even when they are severely immunodeficient clinically; for example, 25% of AIDS patients studied at St Mary's at the time of diagnosis have had T4 numbers within the normal range. This may be explained by the fact that the T4 cells that remain are functionally abnormal — for example, in mitogen responses. T4 lymphocytes show reduced response to their monokine activator interleukin-1 and to their lymphokine growth factor interleukin-2. Production of IL-2 and gamma-interferon by

T4 cells is also reduced. Responses to the T cell mitogens PHA and Concanavalin A and to antigens such as PPD are also defective. T8 cells apparently have normal suppressor function. This serves to emphasise the point that numerical and functional abnormalities of T4 cells are characteristic of AIDS.

B Lymphocytes and Antibodies

B cells are also functionally abnormal, although they are present in normal numbers. This is apparent as a polyclonal rise in gamma-globulin levels (IgG and IgA). It reflects a non-specific stimulation of antibody production to previously encountered antigens and results in raised levels of antibodies to such antigens. Furthermore, they cannot produce an antibody response to a new antigen. These changes may pose problems in the use of serology in diagnostic testing of AIDS patients. Response to stimulation with B cell mitogens such as pokeweed mitogen (T-cell-dependent) and *Staphylococcus aureus* (T-cell-independent) is typically impaired. The polyclonal B cell activation is also responsible for a high prevalence of immune complexes in AIDS patients.

Natural Killer Cells

The functional activity of natural killer cells is reduced in AIDS patients, but phenotypic markers for them (Leu7 and Leu11) give apparently contradictory results. Whether it is a primary defect or is secondary to changes in T cells or reduced interferon production is uncertain. Interferons regulate the production and functional activity of natural killer cells. In addition to reduced gamma-interferon, alpha-interferon production is abnormal. However, increased quantities of an acid-labile form of alpha-interferon, which may be functionally abnormal, are produced. The defect in natural killer cells, which are thought to be involved in the elimination of virus-infected and tumour cells, may provide a clue to the pathogenesis of Kaposi's sarcoma and B cell lymphomas.

Monocytes/Macrophages

Monocyte numbers are reduced. Their function in chemotaxis, adherence and phagocytosis is also abnormal in most AIDS patients. Production of interleukin-1, the lymphocyte-activating monokine, by monocytes may be reduced, although the evidence is conflicting. Killing of intracellular pathogens by macrophages, which are derived from monocytes, is defective but this appears to be largely due to the failure of T4 cells to produce macrophage-activating lymphokines; when exogenous gamma-interferon is provided, the capacity to kill intracellular parasites is restored. On delayed-type hypersensitivity skin testing, AIDS patients show anergy, which also reflects the failure of T cell–macrophage co-operation; this is also shown by their inability to form granulomas with mycobacterial infection. There are no consistent defects in neutrophils or in antibody-dependent cytotoxic responses. Induction of cytotoxic lymphocyte responses is functionally abnormal but this is probably secondary to changes in T4 cells.

Immunogenetics

Early immunogenetic studies on patients with Kaposi's sarcoma showed an increased prevalence of HLA DR5. This HLA antigen is also increased among patients with classical Kaposi's sarcoma, as seen in elderly persons of Ashkenazy Jewish or Mediterranean background. The association between Kaposi's sarcoma and DR5 in AIDS appears to be restricted to persons of this ethnic background. There are as yet no studies on immunogenetic associations with susceptibility to HTLV-III infection or its various clinical expressions.

Diagnostic Tests in AIDS

The characteristic immunological features of AIDS are shown in Table 2.1; they are divided into those that may be available in diagnostic laboratories and those shown by research studies to be of pathogenetic significance. The key features are lymphopenia, an absolute reduction in T4 'helper' cells, polyconal hypergammaglobulinaemia and cutaneous anergy. Like most other laboratory tests, they only have a diagnostic role in defined clinical settings. It is vital to recognise that they are essentially non-specific tests and, even when taken as a group, cannot be used to make a diagnosis of AIDS without clinical evidence of opportunist infections or tumours. This is because similar changes may be seen in unrelated disorders, many of which are seen in at-risk groups; they are also seen in other less severe responses to HTLV-III infection (see below). The diagnosis of AIDS rests on the recognition of a pattern including appropriate clinical and laboratory features. There is considerable variability in the expression of these characterising abnormalities; not all patients show all the features, despite a clear clinical diagnosis of AIDS. The defects are less severe in patients with isolated Kaposi's sarcoma.

Thus, a diagnosis of AIDS is not made, and cannot be made, in the laboratory. In many patients the firm identification of an opportunist infection or tumour is sufficient for diagnosis. This can be backed up by the laboratory findings of lymphopenia and reduced T helper count, together with polyclonal hypergammaglobulinaemia and anergy to several recall antigens. If any of these are normal, it does not necessarily exclude the diagnosis. Laboratory studies are more helpful in patients in whom some doubt exists as to the clinical evidence for immunodeficiency. Finding the typical profile of AIDS may be a guide to how the patient should be regarded operationally, but still cannot be a basis for diagnosis in isolation. In some such instances, judgement on diagnosis should be reserved and the current clinical problems handled according to their immediate priorities. In due course the diagnosis will become evident from careful clinical monitoring. Although the uncertainty may be difficult for both patient and doctor, it is

Table 2.1 Laboratory abnormalities in AIDS

Commonly available assays	Other important changes
Lymphopenia (T cell)*	
T4 (helper) depletion*	
	T4, Leu8 depletion
Reduced mitogen responses	
Reduced antigen responses	
	Defective T4 help in Ig production
	Decreased IL-2 production
	Decreased response to IL-2
	Decreased gamma-IFN production
Anergy to DTH antigens*	
Monocytopenia	
	Monocyte locomotor defect
	Monocyte phagocytic defect
Reduced NK function	
Increased Leu7	
Decreased Leu11	
Polyclonal rise in Igs*	
	Increased spontaneous Ig production
	Decreased B cell mitogen response
	Reduced Ig response to neoantigen
Circulating immune complexes	
Raised acid-labile alpha-IFN	
Raised beta-2 microglobulin	

* = characterising abnormalities, especially in combination.
IFN = interferon.

preferable to making an unsubstantiated diagnosis of AIDS. Some of the problems of diagnostic testing in other HTLV-III-related conditions and among apparently healthy members of risk groups will be discussed below. In many cases the management of the patient — and the relevance of laboratory tests, in particular — should be discussed with a clinical immunologist or equivalent specialist.

HTLV-III Antibodies in Clinical Diagnosis

Considerable care is needed in using HTLV-III antibodies in the diagnosis of AIDS, and indeed in the diagnosis of anything.

The presence of such antibodies simply confirms that a person has been infected by the HTLV-III virus, but, if HTLV-III-positive, cannot determine whether or not any clinical disorder is due to that virus. If positive in a patient who obviously has AIDS and is at risk for contracting HTLV-III, antibodies have added nothing. However, among high-risk groups, who are now commonly seropositive and in whom the diagnosis of AIDS may need to be considered, it may be hard to establish a causal relationship between non-specific symptoms and HTLV-III serology; this is especially true in the absence of previously recognised features that are typical of AIDS or a related disorder. A positive result in someone with definite AIDS who is not apparently at high risk for this infection makes it likely that the immunodeficiency is due to the retrovirus; it may have other important consequences, but largely from the perspective of an infectious disease.

If HTLV-III antibodies are negative in a patient with clinical AIDS, especially if the patient is in a high-risk group, the negative may be false; a decline in HTLV-III antibody levels until they are undetectable has been seen as AIDS develops or progresses, and is due to general failure of humoral immunity. Therefore, one would be inclined to ignore such a result. On the other hand, if a patient has several possible reasons for being immunodeficient, a negative test might sway one in favour of an alternative cause. This may be particularly applicable to a patient who is not from a high-risk group, where HTLV-III-induced immune deficiency enters into the differential diagnosis. Many of the same arguments can be rehearsed for other disorders in which HTLV-III is implicated.

IMMUNOPATHOGENESIS

The Biological Nature of the Immunodeficiency

The clear identification of HTLV-III as the retrovirus responsible for AIDS has brought work on immunopathogenesis into sharper focus. From a pathogenetic point of view, the cardinal defects are the reduced numbers and defective function of T4 lymphocytes; these account for most of the observed abnormalities, so that they are the most obvious candidates for direct viral damage. Functional abnormalities in monocytes/macrophages, natural killer cells, cytotoxic T cells and B cells could in principle be either primary or a consequence of defective T4 cell function. However, from analogies with other immunodeficiencies it seems likely that the primary defect is due to more than just a defect of T cells. This is because the biological immune defect is evidently more profound than that seen in the Di George syndrome − the prototype T cell immunodeficiency; it is more closely analogous to severe combined immune deficiency, a stem cell disorder affecting both T and B cells. In AIDS, combined defects affecting primarily T and B cells or T cells and macrophages would seem probable.

Specific Properties of HTLV-III in Relation to the Immune System

The human retroviruses so far identified appear to be distinguished by their effects on T lymphocytes, particularly T4 cells; HTLV-I leads to transformation of T4 cells, although it may infect other cell types. Recent evidence has shown that HTLV-III has a specific tropism for the same cells, the T4 antigen being an essential part of the virus receptor. Thus, HTLV-III not only attacks the cells of the immune system, but also uses a part of their intrinsic communications system as its receptor. This has a notable parallel with the mouse LDH virus, which uses MHC Class II antigens as receptors, these antigens being complementary to T4 in the language of the immune system. HTLV-III is a cytopathic virus and does not show transforming ability. The nature of the cytopathic effects *in vivo* is unknown but it may involve either lysis or less severe damage followed by reticulo-endothelial clearance.

Relationship between HTLV-III and the Biological Defects

If only those cells that bear the T4 antigen can be infected, primary immuno-pathogenetic mechanisms must again focus on the T4 lymphocyte. All the evidence from patients confirms that these cells are reduced in number and function. However, it is known that some macrophages and related cells also bear the T4 antigen, which explains some of the intrinsic defects seen in these cells. It is probable that the brain cells that are infected by HTLV-III, giving rise to the 'AIDS encephalopathy', are T4-positive microglia. Can B cells be directly infected as well? It has been possible to infect Epstein–Barr virus (EBV)-transformed lymphocytes *in vitro*, but this may reflect the fact that some such cells bear T4 antigen. This may or may not be a feature of EBV-transformed B cells *in vivo*. Alternatively, polyclonal B cell activation could be a non-specific effect of viral infection and is seen with other infectious agents. Defects of natural killer cells are not readily explained by direct infection, as they do not bear the T4 antigen, but could be explained as secondary consequences of T4 lympho-cyte and macrophage defects. However, it is a moot point to ask: what is the most sensitive marker for T4, HTLV-III infection or monoclonal antibodies?

Co-factors that may Determine HTLV-III Expression as Disease

Virus replication can be stimulated *in vitro* by activation of infected lympho-cytes – for example, by mitogen or antigen. This has led to the idea that inter-current events which activate T4 cells *in vivo* could have a similar effect. Thus, waves of viral replication would occur during infection, or with other stimuli such as exposure to foreign (allo-) antigen, leading to infection of an increasing proportion of target cells. The loss of a critical proportion of T4-bearing cells would ultimately result in overt immunodeficiency.

Collateral evidence for this hypothesis is given by the differing latent periods between infection and disease in different risk groups. Homosexual men and intravenous drug abusers, who are likely to activate T cells frequently, have a latent period of from 9 months to a year. For transfusion-associated cases and some heterosexual contacts, it may be between 2 and 5 years; these subjects would have less frequent infections. Neonates will also activate T4 cells repeatedly while acquiring their specific immunological repertoire; the latent period for them is 6-12 months. For this reason, many feel that sero-positive subjects should be counselled that they should take steps to minimise their exposure to intercurrent infection, notably sexually transmitted viral infections.

IMMUNOLOGICAL RESPONSES TO HTLV-III INFECTION

Immunological Changes during Viral Infections

The early response to many viral infections is a lymphocytosis due to an increase in lymphocytes of the T8 suppressor/cytotoxic type; there may also be a slight decrease in T4 cells. Such changes are seen with, for example, EBV, CMV, herpes simplex, herpes zoster and hepatitis B virus infections, several of which commonly affect subjects at risk for AIDS. The changes seen in response to such infections must not be confused with those seen in AIDS, nor should they be regarded necessarily as evidence of immunosuppression. The T8 cell increase probably reflects recruitment of cytotoxic cells and seems an appropriate response.

Early Changes in HTLV-III Infection

What happens after HTLV-III infection? An acute glandular-fever-like illness has been seen in some patients in association with seroconversion to HTLV-III; it is accompanied by an increase in T8 lymphocytes. Symptom-free subjects who have been infected with HTLV-III may be normal or may show one of two generally distinct responses — a T8 rise or a T4 fall; these may be transient or may persist. They are not readily distinguishable from the changes following intercurrent events such as other viral infections, which may occur before or after HTLV-III seroconversion.

Changes in PGL and Prodromal AIDS (ARC)

Patients with persistent generalised lymphadenopathy (PGL) show the same two types of immunological change. Some patients show transiently or persistently elevated T8 lymphocyte counts; in others, a fall in T4 cells continues or develops, sometimes transiently. In some subjects studied longitudinally, development of PGL was accompanied by normalisation of previously abnormal lymphocyte sub-set results. These diverse changes confirm the heterogeneous nature of PGL.

Patients with prodromal AIDS (or AIDS-related complex) show T4 lymphocyte depletion which resembles and turns into the typical changes of AIDS itself. Patients with PGL who progress to AIDS tend to have similar symptoms and may show a progressive fall in T4 cells. The various responses seen in subjects who have been infected by HTLV-III could represent either a sequence of changes or different types of response. They could, in turn, reflect differing host susceptibility, the presence or absence of infective or other co-factors; equally, they may herald different outcomes.

Recent work has shown that immunohistological investigation of patients with PGL may provide further evidence of heterogeneity within PGL, which seems relevant to outcome. Patients with associated 'prodromal' symptoms, including several who went on to develop AIDS, showed a characteristic loss of the normal cellular structure of germinal centres in lymph nodes. This structure is normally maintained by follicular dendritic reticular (FDR) cells and patients with destruction of the FDR structure of germinal centres have a worse prognosis. There was no direct relationship between the FDR cell changes and T4 lymphocyte numbers.

Why T Cell 'Ratios' are Unhelpful

Many authors have reported data on peripheral blood lymphocyte sub-sets as T4/T8, 'helper/suppressor', ratios. This may have seemed a convenient formulation for non-immunologists, but it has no evident biological significance. More importantly, it has thoroughly obscured the two distinct responses to HTLV-III infection. With T4 cells as the target for retrovirus-induced damage and T8 cells as potential responders to it, as well as to unrelated infections, there seems little sense in combining separate measures into a figure that no longer distinguishes them.

Diagnostic Immunology in HTLV-III Risk Subjects

It will be apparent from the foregoing that the immunological markers for AIDS may resemble the changes seen in other intercurrent events in high-risk patients, such as sexually active homosexual males and haemophiliacs. Indeed, longitudinal studies have shown that T4 depletion and T8 increase are commonly seen as transient events in these populations in the absence of HTLV-III infection, apparently in response to intercurrent infections and possibly other events. Anergy to DTH skin tests is also common in such populations. Polyclonal B cell activation may occur in response to a number of non-specific B cell activators that may occur during various infections and on allogeneic stimulation.

In patients with PGL and prodromal AIDS, lymphocyte sub-set testing may be helpful in broadly identifying those with persistent T4 cell depletion, who are more likely to be truly prodromal for AIDS. But in symptom-free subjects, even those who are known to be HTLV-III-antibody-positive, these changes may not be related to this retrovirus infection; this is especially true if the changes are transient. Their predictive role in defining those most likely to progress to symptomatic infection with HTLV-III has yet to be established. There is therefore little justification for screening tests of this type in a well person. Only the presence of clinical problems that are clearly related to the retrovirus can justify their use. Even in such individuals, their interpretation is difficult, and longitudinal study is more helpful than single observations. The evaluation of such tests in long-term cohort studies is under way, and their role should be clarified in due course.

Protective Immunity to HTLV-III

What protective immune responses can develop against HTLV-III? In principle, these are likely to be of two forms: neutralising antibody and cytotoxic T cells. It is clear that the detectable antibody is not protective, being found in well and ill alike; neutralising activity appears to be low. The lack of neutralising antibodies may be important in not limiting free viraemia and, hence, in determining infectivity. However, on basic principles, elimination of virally infected cells is more likely to be achieved by cytotoxic T cells. It is important to establish what, if any, protective immune responses do occur as a background to the development of vaccines.

APPROACHES TO TREATMENT AND PREVENTION

Immune Reconstitution

Knowing the pathogenetic mechanism for the immunodeficiency should facilitate a directed approach to therapy. So far, clinical benefit from attempted immune reconstitution has been negligible. The logical approach is bone marrow transplantation, to restore the parts of the immune system that have been destroyed. It is effective in reconstitution of severe combined immunodeficiency. Attempts so far have been unsuccessful, presumably because the new T4 cells were reinfected by persisting retrovirus. Combining long-term antiviral therapy with bone marrow transplantation may be a future option.

An alternative approach to the treatment of AIDS would be to replace those factors that T4 lymphocytes produce, and lymphokine reconstitution of this sort is still being evaluated, generally as single-agent systemic therapy. Interleukin-2 and gamma-interferon (both natural product and recombinant types) have been used individually, but show negligible clinical efficacy despite some *in vitro* improvement. A combination would seem more logical but has not yet been evaluated. IL-2 could in theory, by stimulating lymphocyte proliferation, enhance virus replication in latently infected cells. This is perhaps of most concern in less severe variants of HTLV-III infection, in which T4 cells are not already depleted.

Macrophage-activating lymphokines other than gamma-interferon are not yet characterised, but could be essential to the success of this strategy.

The efficacy of alpha-interferon in some patients with Kaposi's sarcoma can be regarded as a form of immune reconstitution, enhancing the production/ function of natural killer cells in patients who retain sufficient function. Thymic factors and transplants have shown no convincing evidence of efficacy, but may find a role as a part of combination therapy. Isoprinosine (Imunovir) is ineffective in AIDS but appears to show some promise in PGL, where it may lead to increased T cell levels and natural killer function. It is too early to say whether or not these functional changes are biologically significant.

Antiviral Therapy against HTLV-III

It seems likely that any future strategy will need to include antiviral therapy, especially in view of the encephalopathy, which is clearly independent of effects on the immune system, but also to ensure that remaining cells or new cells are not reinfected. Whether the administration of lymphokine cocktails or bone marrow transplantation emerges as the immunorestorative method of choice remains to be seen. Intervention earlier in disease will depend more on the use of effective antivirals and on stimulating function in the cells that remain.

Vaccines

The development of a safe and effective vaccine is likely to take some time and is already posing a number of problems. The need to promote a protective immune response implies a knowledge of what protective responses are effective. The stimulation of antibody and cytotoxic lymphocyte responses may require different viral antigens. The variability of the envelope protein among most isolates indicates possible problems in this approach. When a vaccine does become available, many of the current high-risk groups will be already infected — it is interesting to consider who should receive a vaccine.

Protective Measures before Vaccines are Available

However, there is still much prevention to be done which can reduce the spread of HTLV-III infection and minimise its effects in those who are already infected. The vast majority of AIDS cases are sexually transmitted, with a substantial number caused by sharing of equipment by intravenous drug abusers. Risk reduction through minimising numbers of sexual, especially casual, partners among both homosexuals and heterosexuals, and by using safe sex methods (including use of condoms), where risk is high, are especially important. Attempts to reduce unsafe practices among intravenous drug abusers may be more difficult to achieve in practice, but common-sense dictates that the mixing of blood should be avoided. These measures are important not only in reducing exposure to the retrovirus for those not yet infected, but also in reducing exposure to other infections that may activate T4 cells in HTLV-III-infected subjects, enhancing virus replication and damaging the immune system to the point of immunodeficiency.

CONCLUSIONS

AIDS has posed many challenges for medicine, science and society. As an immunodeficiency disease, it has clarified many basic concepts of immunology, both scientifically and diagnostically. The epidemiology of the disease led naturally to the concept that it resulted from an infectious agent, probably a virus. Its biological properties could again be deduced from clinical and epidemiological evidence, and strongly favoured a retrovirus; this led to the identification of HTLV-III. The elucidation of the pathogenesis followed swiftly on from the demonstration of the aetiological agent; this was greatly facilitated by the large amount of data already collected on immunological changes in AIDS patients. The cellular immune defect seen indicated a highly specific effect of the virus on certain parts of the immune system. The role of the T4 antigen as the HTLV-III receptor illustrates a remarkable mechanism in viral immunopathology, and one which has a notable analogy in the LDH virus of mice: that is to say, the use by a virus of one of the key communication signals in the immune system. Thus, all the key discoveries about AIDS have been derived from careful clinical and epidemiological studies, which emphasises the central importance of clinical observation and of patients themselves as a base for scientific research into human disease.

The role of diagnostic immunology in AIDS is important, but only in a defined clinical context; indeed, clinical assessment remains the backbone of management. In patients with other variants of HTLV-III infection, such as PGL and prodromal AIDS, immunological investigation does seem to have a role in identifying subjects at higher risk of developing AIDS. The relevance of T cell sub-set testing and other immunological screening in asymptomatic members of high-risk populations is far from clear, and remains a subject for research study; longitudinal observation is more likely to be of value than single 'snapshots', which are likely to be confounded by other events. However, no amount of laboratory immunology can substitute for good clinical judgement.

BIBLIOGRAPHY

Bowen, D. L., Lane, H. C. and Fauci, A. S. (1984). Cellular immunity. In Ebbesen, P., Biggar, R. J. and Melbye, M. (Eds.), *AIDS — A Basic Guide for Clinicians*, pp. 135–150. Munksgaard, Copenhagen

Cooper, D. A., Gold, J., Maclean, P., Donovan, B., Finlayson, R., Barnes, T. G., Michelmore, H. M., Brooke, P. and Penny, R. (1985). Acute AIDS-retrovirus infection — definition of a clinical illness associated with seroconversion. *Lancet*, **i**, 537

Janossy, G., Pinching, A. J., Bofill, M., Weber, J., McLaughlin, J. E., Ornstein, M., Ivory, K., Harris, J. R. W., Favrot, M. and Macdonald-Burns, D. C. (1985). An immunohistological approach to persistent lymphadenopathy and its relevance to AIDS. *Clin. Exp. Immunol.*, **59**, 257

Lane, H. C., Masur, H., Edgar, L. C., Whalen, G. and Fauci, A. S. (1983). Abnormalities of B lymphocyte activation and immunoregulation in patients with the acquired immunodeficiency syndrome. *New Engl. J. Med.*, **309**, 453

Murray, H. W., Rubin, B. Y., Masur, H. and Roberts, R. B. (1984). Impaired production of lymphokines and immune (gamma) interferon in the acquired immunodeficiency syndrome. *New Engl. J. Med.*, **310**, 883

Pinching, A. J. (1984a). The acquired immune deficiency syndrome. *Clin. Exp. Immunol.*, **56**, 1

Pinching, A. J. (1984b). The immunology of AIDS — Meeting report. *J. Roy. Soc. Med.*, **77**, 971

Pinching, A. J., McManus, T. J., Jeffries, D. J., Moshtael, O., Donaghy, M., Parkin, J. M., Munday, P. E. and Harris, J. R. W. (1983). Studies of cellular immunity in male homosexuals in London. *Lancet*, **ii**, 126

Pinching, A. J. and Weiss, R. A. (1985). AIDS and the spectrum of HTLV-III/LAV infection. *Int. Rev. Exp. Pathol.*, **28** (in press)

Seligmann, M., Chess, L., Fahey, J. L., Fauci, A. S., Lachmann, P. J., L'Age-Stehr, J., Ngu, J., Pinching, A. J., Rosen, P., Spira, T. J. and Wybran, J. (1984). AIDS — An immunologic reevaluation. *New Engl. J. Med.*, **311**, 1286

Zolla-Pazner, S. (1984). Serology. In Ebbesen, P., Biggar, R. J. and Melbye, M. (Eds.), *AIDS — A Basic Guide for Clinicians*, pp. 151–172. Munksgaard, Copenhagen

3
Virology

Don Jeffries

HTLV-III/LAV – A HUMAN RETROVIRUS

AIDS and related conditions have been causally associated with a newly recognised exogenous retrovirus. This virus has been termed lymphadenopathy virus (LAV: Barré-Sinoussi *et al.*, 1983), human T lymphotropic virus type III (HTLV-III: Popovic *et al.*, 1984) and AIDS-associated retrovirus (ARV: Levy *et al.*, 1984). To avoid unnecessary repetition, the abbreviation HTLV-III will be used. Retroviruses contain RNA and use a viral enzyme called reverse transcriptase (RNA-dependent DNA polymerase) to make a DNA copy of their RNA genome. The three main genes of the viruses (*gag-*, *pol-* and *env-*) are flanked by long terminal repeats (LTR) which are responsible for integrating the DNA copy (provirus) into the DNA of host cells. The basic genomic structure of this type of retrovirus is shown in Figure 3.1.

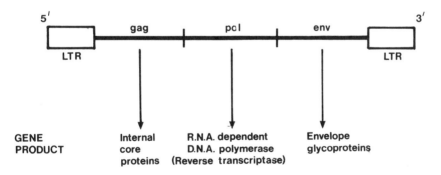

Figure 3.1 Genomic structure of retroviruses

Some animal retroviruses contain a cell-derived DNA sequence (*onc* gene) which allows them to induce acute transformation with rapid onset of malignancy in their host species. Others are responsible for a variety of non-malignant conditions, as listed in Table 3.1.

Table 3.1 Retrovirus diseases in animals

Malignancies
  leukaemia
  lymphoma
  carcinoma
  sarcoma
Immune deficiency
Autoimmunity
Osteopetrosis
Slow neuropathy
Pneumonia

HTLV-III does not contain an oncogene and has not been directly linked with malignant transformation. Acquired immune deficiency is, however, a well-recognised effect of other retroviruses — for example, feline leukaemia virus.

Unlike HTLV-I (the retrovirus known to cause T cell leukaemia in humans), which is capable of existing for long periods in the proviral form, HTLV-III establishes a productive infection. This continued virus replication appears to lead to the progressive depletion of the main cell population infected by the virus which are CD4-antigen-bearing (helper) T cells. It is significant that the only cells known to be susceptible to infection with HTLV-III are those possessing this surface antigen — i.e. CD4-positive lymphocytes, antigen-presenting cells (macrophage series) and possibly B lymphocytes under certain conditions (e.g. Epstein-Barr-virus-infected). Dalgleish *et al.* (1984) have firmly established that the receptor for the virus is either the CD4 antigen itself or a closely related structure. A scheme for the replication of a productive retrovirus infection is shown in Figure 3.2.

Major milestones in the search for human retroviruses were the discovery of reverse transcriptase by Baltimore (1970) and Temin and Mizutani (1970), followed by the identification and purification of T cell growth factor (TCGF) by Morgan *et al.* (1976). With TCGF it became possible to establish T cell lines from normal individuals and from those with T cell neoplasms. This work resulted in the identification and characterisation of HTLV-I and HTLV-II and ultimately led to the successful cultivation of HTLV-III. HTLV-III has now been isolated from several hundred individuals with AIDS or PGL and also from asymptomatic people with evidence of exposure to the virus as judged by HTLV-III antibody positivity. Use of permissive cell lines for production of high-titre virus has allowed antibody detection systems to be developed.

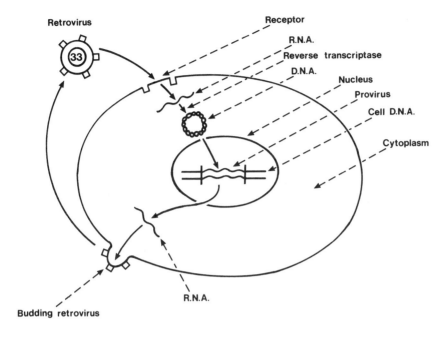

Figure 3.2 Retrovirus replication cycle

LABORATORY DIAGNOSIS OF HTLV-III INFECTION

At present virus culture with confirmation of positivity by reverse transcriptase detection, immunofluorescence and electron microscopy remains a research procedure and is not easily adaptable for routine diagnosis. Because of the low numbers of overtly infected lymphocytes and the low levels of cell-free antigen, there is little prospect of antigen detection assays. In consequence, antibody detection systems offer the most satisfactory approach to routine diagnosis. Several techniques have been described, including enzyme-linked immunosorbent assays (ELISA), radio-immunoassays (RIA), membrane-immunofluorescence, fixed-cell immunofluorescence and Western blotting. ELISA tests are the first to be introduced on a commercial basis.

SIGNIFICANCE OF RESULTS OF ANTIBODY TESTING

Antibody-positive asymptomatic individuals have been shown to transmit HTLV-III by sexual intercourse and blood transfusion. It has also been established that virus can be isolated from people several years after becoming antibody-positive. This means that, until evidence to the contrary is forthcoming, a positive HTLV-III antibody test means that the individual may have a continuing productive infection and must, therefore, be presumed to be potentially infectious to sexual partners and to those receiving his/her blood. Those who are engaged in testing for this antibody must be aware of the profound implications of reporting a positive result.

Now that commercial tests are available, the major problems lie less in the tests themselves than in the careful and time-consuming counselling required by those who convey the result to the individual concerned. These very serious considerations are compounded by the fact that the tests are not totally reliable. By screening large numbers of low-risk sera (i.e. blood donors) the positive rate, and therefore the false-positive rate, is reassuringly low. What is disconcerting, however, is that there is at present no suitable confirmatory test which will allow one to pronounce a 'positive' test by ELISA, RIA or immunofluorescence a true- or false-positive. Western blotting has been recommended for this purpose but has been found to be insufficiently sensitive. 'False-negative' tests also occur, and isolation of viruses from individuals in whom the most sensitive antibody tests are repeatedly negative has been documented. This is all that one might expect from antibody tests which are always second best to virus culture or antigen detection, and, in fact, the first-generation tests are performing remarkably well. All one can do at present is confirm the positive result on a second sample and by more than one test system. If the procedure of virus culture becomes more adaptable to the routine laboratory, confirmation of continuing infection may become easier.

PHYSICOCHEMICAL PROPERTIES OF HTLV-III AND ITS INACTIVATION

Although, at the time of writing, the virus is showing signs of genomic variation, it will always have the characteristic properties of a retrovirus. Long before AIDS first appeared, workers on related animal retroviruses had documented the physicochemical characteristics of viruses in this family (Vogt, 1965). It is reasonable, to an extent, to predict the inactivation characteristics of HTLV-III from this earlier work, and recent data largely confirm these predictions. Retroviruses are surrounded by a lipid-containing membrane, and integrity of this membrane is essential for infectivity. Not surprisingly, therefore, they are susceptible to lipid solvents, and there is already preliminary evidence that infectivity of HTLV-III is abolished by 50% ether, 25% ethanol and 0.5% titron X-100. As one might expect, the virus is inactivated by β-propionolactone (0.1%), formalin 0.1%, paraformaldehyde (0.5%) and 52.5 p.p.m. sodium hypochlorite. These preliminary data were reported at the International Conference on AIDS, Atlanta, Georgia, in April 1985. It must be stressed, however, that although these agents show considerable virucidal activity in test systems, much higher concentrations will be necessary if proteinaceous material is present. It is, therefore, sensible to retain the recommended concentrations of disinfectant present in use for hepatitis B decontamination.

Retroviruses, in general, are very sensitive to heat, and early studies with HTLV-III indicate that this virus is no exception. Several groups have reported total inactivation of the virus following incubation at 56°C for 30 min. Spire *et al*. (1985) have found that this occurs even when the serum concentration is 50%, and they advocate heating under these conditions as a possible way of increasing the safety of handling serum samples in the laboratory. As other workers have described the persistence of some residual infectivity after this treatment, further work is necessary to ensure that the sera may be pronounced totally safe. What is quite clear is that infectivity is rapidly destroyed at higher temperatures, and that boiling and autoclaving are very efficient ways of decontaminating instruments and other materials.

HTLV-III shows the relative resistance to ionising and ultraviolet radiations reported for other retroviruses. Infectivity was retained after exposure to less than 2.5×10^5 rad gamma-rays, and 5×10^3 J/m^2 was required to inactivate the virus by ultraviolet light (Spire *et al*., 1985). These levels are much higher than the emission levels normally employed in safety cabinets and operating theatres.

Data are accumulating rapidly on the exact inactivation characteristics of the virus. This information will be critically important in devising ways of inactivating virus in blood products. The risks to laboratory personnel are, from the epidemiological evidence, exceedingly low, and, on the principle that potential infectivity is dependent on virus titre, any significant reduction in titre may totally eliminate the risk of infection. However, the reader is warned of two pitfalls which may be misleading in attempting to interpret these data. First, the inactivation process may be conducted in a totally artificial situation − e.g. in serum-free tissue culture medium − and thus have no direct relevance to clinical or laboratory practice. Second, the results are only meaningful if the investigators have measured the effects on infectivity, and not on inactivation of a particular virus component such as reverse transcriptase.

CONTROL OF INFECTION WITH HTLV-III

For many months after AIDS was first recognised in the USA, its aetiology, although unknown, was thought to be related to life-style factors, 'antigenic overload' or possibly a variant of a common infectious agent such as cytomegalovirus. For this reason, no special measures were taken to isolate sufferers or those in the risk groups, and samples were handled in routine laboratories. When considering this, one must bear in mind that these patients were given the benefit of all aspects of modern diagnostic techniques which may expose the operator to aerosols and inoculation injury. Despite this lack of stringent precautions, there has not been, at the time of writing, a single case of AIDS in a health care worker anywhere in the world which is attributable to occupational exposure.

t many hundreds of needle injuries have been recorded and
ip, only one individual has developed antibody in circum-
to relate to a known inoculation injury (Anon., 1984). All
evidence points to sexual intercourse, inoculation and trans-
d blood products, and intrauterine infection as being the
on. There is no evidence of spread by aerosols. It is sensible,
t clinical and laboratory practices which are designed to
of blood and other body fluids from a person with evidence
of HTLV-III infection to the health care worker or to other individuals. In this
context, although an ill patient may be harbouring certain opportunist infections
which may present a hazard to others, it is illogical to assume that potential
infectivity of HTLV-III is greater in those with symptoms than in the asymptomatic. Health care personnel are already aware of the measures necessary to
break the transmission chain of serum-borne infections from existing guidelines
for hepatitis B. Inoculation must represent the most important mode of serum
transfer during patient management; and careful handling of needles and sharp
instruments, avoidance of resheathing needles and use of suitable sharps disposal
boxes are important measures to reduce this risk. Glass fragments may present a
similar hazard, and ward and laboratory procedures should be assessed in an
attempt to eliminate or reduce exposure to glass. An apparently intact skin
surface may harbour microcuts and abrasions, and for this reason gloves are
recommended if there is a risk of contact with blood or other body fluids from
a known or suspected HTLV-III-antibody-positive individual. The membranes
of the eyes and mouth may be more permeable to virus particles, and, where
there is a risk of splashing of potentially infectious material, eye and mouth
protection (either a visor or goggles and mask) should be worn.

The principles outlined above form the basis of published guidelines for
patient care and clinical and laboratory investigations. Guidelines have been issued
by the Centres for Disease Control, Atlanta, Georgia, and National Institutes of
Health, Bethesda, Maryland (CDC/NIH, 1982); the University of California, San
Francisco, AIDS task force (Conte *et al.*, 1983); and the Advisory Committee on
Dangerous Pathogens, UK (1984). On the basis of these documents, it is sensible
to produce in-house guidelines which are directly related to local conditions and
practices. As all available epidemiological evidence indicates that HTLV-III
presents little (if any) risk to health care staff or to other individuals except by
the recognised transmission routes, safety precautions should be scientifically
justifiable and not excessively stringent to handicap normal management and
investigation of patients.

Isolation of Patients

Isolation of patients with HTLV-III infection may be desirable for several
reasons. With a virus which is immunosuppressive, a case could be made for protective isolation if the patient requires in-patient care. However, in view of the

fact that there is little evidence that the common opportunist organisms are nosocomially acquired, this is probably not a significant factor in management. Source isolation may be considered for two reasons. First, if the patient is infected with one of the few recognised opportunist agents which present a risk to others, isolation may be required until the infection has been controlled. Second, although there is no evidence that HTLV-III is transmissible other than by transfer of body fluids, a case can be made for regarding some patients as 'higher-risk'. Haematemesis, multiple wounds, and profuse and frequent diarrhoea are examples of complicating factors where the exposure to body fluids is likely to be greater than in most other patients — e.g. those with Kaposi's sarcoma or with CNS problems.

Laboratory Precautions

The principles outlined in the introduction to this section should also be applied in the transportation, reception and processing of all samples from confirmed or suspected HTLV-III-antibody-positive individuals. Although there is no evidence that aerosol transmission occurs, procedures such as virus culture, which are calculated to amplify the infectivity of the virus or which expose the operator to higher than normal airborne concentrations, should be performed in a suitable safety cabinet. By giving careful consideration to eliminating potential sources of inoculation injury — e.g. needles, glass pasteur pipettes, cover slips, etc. — working conditions can be made very much safer. In the UK, laboratory staff wish to have notification of samples from HTLV-III-antibody-positive individuals. This is achieved by applying an alerting label (often the international biohazard symbol) to the form and specimen container. It can be argued that this system is beneficial in allowing 'higher-risk' samples to be handled under appropriate levels of containment and that this leads to a reduction of risks. The argument is tenable provided that the laboratory staff are fully aware that there is no implication that the unmarked samples are safe. Unless HTLV-III antibody testing becomes very extensive, there is a considerable possibility that more positive sera will be handled in the unmarked sera than in those hazard-labelled, quite apart from potential risks from other viruses, such as hepatitis B and non-A non-B, which may also be present.

Health Surveillance

In the interim guidelines produced by the Advisory Committee on Dangerous Pathogens (1984) in the UK, the following recommendations are made: 'Those who may be directly exposed to the body fluids and tissues of AIDS patients and those undertaking laboratory work on viable HTLV-III should be asked to volunteer [sic] serum samples. These should be taken before starting work and at six monthly intervals thereafter and be kept in long-term storage. Arrangements should be made to test these sera for the presence of HTLV-III antibody and the results recorded as part of a surveillance scheme.'

Anyone who considers implementing such a scheme should, as with any laboratory testing, think through the consequences of finding a positive result. If a staff member is found to be positive, either on the first serum or subsequently, the result is likely to have a profound influence on his/her personal life. It is to be hoped that further work will inform us that antibody does not necessarily indicate continuing infectivity, but at present one must assume that this test suggests the possibility of infecting sexual partners and recipients of blood donations. The 'positive' may be a false positive. While there is no confirmatory test, some individuals are in danger of being wrongly labelled positive and, therefore, potentially infectious. Staff members should consider the possible prejudices and implications for other aspects of their professional life. This may be particularly relevant to those employed in dentistry, surgery and, possibly, haemodialysis units. Thought should also be given to the implications of HTLV-III positivity in the context of applications for life insurance.

The guidelines issued by the ACDP are commendable in terms of gathering information on risks (or absence of risks) to health care staff. They have little to offer, apart from worry, for the staff members involved. Unless an employer, who has thought through the implications, seriously wants HTLV-III testing, the following approach may be more satisfactory.

(1) All staff working with HTLV-III-positive individuals, or materials from them, should be given the opportunity to provide a serum sample.
(2) This sample should be stored indefinitely in a locked deep freezer (at −40°C or less), not removed or tested for any reason without the knowledge and permission of the person concerned.
(3) Illness during the person's period of employment should be reported to the occupational health physician or alternative medical adviser.
(4) If it is considered that the stored baseline serum would assist in the diagnosis of a particular disease, it may be released and tested together with later sera, with the knowledge and permission of the staff member concerned. It should be determined by consultation between the virologist, occupational health physician and staff member concerned exactly which tests will be performed and whether HTLV-III antibody tests are necessary.

Inoculation Injuries

There are certain first aid measures, dictated by common-sense, which should be applied to inoculation injuries. These are as follows: (1) encourage bleeding at the puncture site; (2) wash liberally with soap and water; (3) report to the person responsible for the work; (4) report the incident to the occupational health physician (if appropriate).

The recommended procedure from that stage depends on the views of that particular unit. The policy operated by some is to conduct regular medical examinations accompanied by testing for HTLV-III antibody. The reader must decide whether this system, which is ideal for gathering epidemiological information, is in the best interests of the individual. An alternative approach (that favoured by the author) is to take a baseline serum which is stored under the same security arrangements as those described in the previous section. The staff member is then offered a brief six-monthly medical consultation to ensure that health is maintained, and no further samples are taken unless a clinical indication arises.

Public Health Aspects

As knowledge of HTLV-III infection and AIDS increases, it will, it is hoped, be possible to identify relevant co-factors which are contributing to the progressive immune deficiency. When this is the case, counselling of those in the risk groups will become more definitive and based less on calculated guesswork. Some measures are logical and sensible, and these are discussed in Chapter 11. Condoms have been shown to satisfactorily exclude certain infectious agents — e.g. herpes simplex and *Chlamydia* — in experimental systems and might reasonably be expected to offer an impermeable barrier to retroviruses or infected lymphocytes.

At the time of writing there is a firm intention to introduce routine HTLV-III antibody screening of blood donors in the UK. In view of the fact that false negatives are likely, this screening process must be combined with a continuation of the recommendation that those in recognised risk groups should not donate blood. Blood donor screening should also reduce the risks of contamination of factor VIII concentrate and other blood products. Again, however, because of the risk of false negatives, heat treatment will probably have to continue to ensure that any virus in the final pools is inactivated. It has been stated that widespread testing of individuals in the risk groups must be introduced in parallel with the donor screening. The reason given is that, unless antibody testing is freely available, there will be a tendency for those at risk to enrol as blood donors to determine their antibody status.

The ethical issues surrounding the introduction of this test are profound. These problems are discussed by Osterholm *et al.* (1985). Some have argued that it is the blood recipient who requires protection and that the donors should not be informed. This would mean that the transfusion centre would be party to information about an individual which may have serious or fatal implications for the individual's sexual partner(s) and possibly children. It is surely ethically unacceptable to withhold this information. Blood donor screening and testing of people in risk groups will reveal an increasing number of antibody-positives. Provision must be made for staff with the ability and time to offer adequate guidance and counselling to these people.

CONCLUSION

In conclusion, one must stress that knowledge is being gathered with encouraging speed. It remains to be seen whether control of HTLV-III infection can be assisted by vaccines or antiviral drugs. However, it is difficult to imagine that, in the foreseeable future, the world will become 'AIDS-free'. There are many unanswered problems. It is better to tackle these problems carefully and singly, but inevitably there is considerable pressure to find solutions sooner rather than later. Ideally it would have been sensible to spend longer assessing HTLV-III antibody testing systems before introducing them without a confirmatory test. Time will tell us the implications of HTLV-III in dialysis units, in organ grafting and in women in pregnancy.

This chapter is designed to raise some of the important issues which need to be considered by those coping with the practical problems of AIDS. It is not intended to produce yet another set of guidelines, but it is hoped that these comments will assist people in implementing the existing recommendations sensibly and on scientific grounds.

BACKGROUND READING

Weiss, R., Teich, N. and Coffin, J. (1984). *R.N.A. Tumour Viruses*. Cold Spring Harbour Laboratory

REFERENCES

Advisory Committee on Dangerous Pathogens (1984). *AIDS – Interim Guidelines*. HSE/DHSS, London

Anon. (1984). Needlestick transmission of HTLV-III from a patient infected in Africa. *Lancet*, **ii**, 1376

Baltimore, D. (1970). Viral R.N.A.-dependent DNA polymerase. *Nature, Lond.*, **226**, 1209

Barré-Sinoussi, F., Chermann, J. C., Rey, F., Nugeyre, M. T., Chamaret, S., Gruest, J., Danguet, C., Axler-Blin, C., Venizet-Brun, F., Rouzioux, C., Rosenbaum, W. and Montagnier, L. (1983). Isolation of T lymphotropic retrovirus from a patient at risk for acquired immune deficiency syndrome (AIDS). *Science, N.Y.*, **220**, 868

CDC/NIH (1982). Acquired Immune Deficiency Syndrome (AIDS): Precautions for clinical and laboratory staffs. *Morbidity and Mortality Weekly Record*, **31**, 577

Conte, J. E., Hadley, W. K., Sande, M. and the University of California, San Francisco, Task Force on Acquired Immunodeficiency Syndrome (1983).

Infection Control Guidelines for patients with the acquired immunodeficiency syndrome (AIDS). *New Engl. J. Med.*, **309**, 740

Dalgleish, A. G., Beverley, P. C. L., Clapham, P. R., Crawford, D. H., Greaves, M. F. and Weiss, R. A. (1984). The CD4 (T4) antigen is an essential component of the receptor for the AIDS retrovirus. *Nature, Lond.*, **312**, 763

Levy, J. A., Hoffman, A. D., Kramer, S. M., Landis, J. A., Shimabuburo, J. M. and Oshiro, L. S. (1984). Isolation of lympocytopathic retroviruses from San Francisco patients with AIDS. *Science, N.Y.*, **255**, 840

Morgan, D. A., Ruscetti, F. W. and Gallo, R. (1976). Selective in vitro growth of T lymphocytes from normal human bone marrows. *Science, N.Y.*, **193**, 1007

Osterholm, M. T., Bowman, R. J., Chopek, M. W., McCullogh, J. J., Korlath, J. A. and Polesky, H. F. (1985). Screening donated blood and plasma for HTLV-III antibody: Facing more than one crisis? *New Engl. J. Med.*, **312**, 1185

Popovic, M., Sarngadharan, M. G., Read, E. and Gallo, R. C. (1984). Detection, isolation and continuous production of cytopathic retroviruses (HTLV-III) from patients with AIDS and pre-AIDS. *Science, N.Y.*, **224**, 497

Spire, B., Barré-Sinoussi, F., Chermann, J. D., Dormont, D. and Montagnier, L. (1985). Inactivation of lymphadenopathy-associated virus by heat, gamma rays, and ultraviolet light. *Lancet*, **i**, 188

Temin, H. M. and Mizutani, S. (1970). RNA-dependent DNA polymerase in virions of Rous sarcoma virus. *Nature, Lond.*, **226**, 1211

Vogt, P. K. (1965). Avian tumor viruses. *Adv. Virus Res.*, **11**, 293

4
Venereology

Greta Forster

INTRODUCTION

The first case of AIDS in the United Kingdom was reported in December 1981 (Dubois *et al.*, 1981). By May 1985, 169 patients fulfilled the CDC epidemiological case definition of AIDS, with 78 deaths. The exponential rise continues with doubling of reported cases every 8 months.

A majority of AIDS cases (88%) have occurred in homosexual or bisexual men, who may comprise 6% of adult males. However, the total number of homosexual men in the UK is unknown (Green and Miller, 1985). HTLV-III infection has become well established since 1980 among those homosexuals who have attended departments of genito-urinary medicine (GUM) in Britain (Mortimer *et al.*, 1985). A proportion of these will later develop AIDS-related diseases. Heterosexual transmission of HTLV-III infection has been reported from Central Africa and may become important among drug abusers and haemophiliacs.

Guidelines on the clinical presentation and diagnosis of HTLV-III infection have been circulated to all doctors in England (DHSS, 1985). Referral of suspected cases to departments of GUM is advised. This chapter outlines the organisation and facilities of the sexually transmitted diseases (STD) service in the UK. Recommendations for the management of patients presenting with HTLV-III infection or AIDS concern, are based upon our clinical experience at St Mary's Hospital, London. The Praed Street Clinic is the largest department of GUM in Britain, seeing some 40 000 new out-patients each year, of whom 25% are homosexual or bisexual men. Our knowledge is representative of that gained within the larger STD clinics in central London, but cannot be considered typical of all departments in the UK.

THE STD SERVICE IN THE UNITED KINGDOM

Development

Local authorities were required by the *Venereal Disease Regulations* of 1916 to provide free and confidential treatment for all persons suffering from venereal diseases. These were based on the recommendations of a Royal Commission set up in 1913 to report on the prevalence and consequences of venereal diseases (classified as syphilis, gonorrhoea and chancroid). The *Venereal Disease Act* of 1917 provided greater protection for patients by restricting treatment to registered medical practitioners. A comprehensive network of clinics developed, and was integrated into the National Health Service when this was established in 1948. The speciality of genito-urinary medicine has evolved, representing changing patterns in sexually transmitted diseases (Catterall, 1984).

Organisation

The population of the UK (estimated at 56 million in 1982) is served by 230 departments of GUM. Thirty of some 180 clinics in England are based in Greater London. Half of all new cases of STD were looked after by the four Thames regions in 1983 (Anon., 1985). The majority of HTLV-III infection and AIDS cases have also been seen in these departments.

One consultant in GUM for every half-million population is recommended by the Department of Health. In 1983 there were 115 consultants in post. The physician is supported by junior staff in training, hospital practitioners and clinical assistants. Ancillary staff contribute to the clinic team, and include nurses, health advisers, receptionists and secretaries. Few departments have access to their own in-patient beds, but will utilise medical, gynaecological or dermatological wards as individually appropriate.

All residents of the UK and visitors who stay in the country for more than 24 h have free access to the clinics: no referral letter is required. An appointment system may be in use but will be waived for urgent consultations. Free and confidential facilities are provided for the investigation, diagnosis and treatment of patients who suspect that they may have acquired a sexually transmitted infection.

Sexually Transmitted Diseases

After World War II venereal diseases were considered to be in decline because of a reduction in cases of syphilis and gonorrhoea. However, the prevalence of other STD increased steadily by 5–10% per annum from the mid-1950s. Non-specific genital infection became notifiable in 1951. The present diagnostic categories, including herpes simplex virus infection and genital warts, were introduced in 1972. Over 500 000 new cases were recorded for the first time in 1980, other conditions requiring and not requiring treatment forming the largest diagnostic category. These statistics are based on the annual returns, completed by physicians in charge of clinics, and published each year in the Annual Report of the Chief Medical Officer of the Department of Health and Social Security.

Sexual transmission of AIDS and HTLV-III infection has been recognised in the majority of cases. However, clinic returns have not been revised to include these diagnostic categories, and they are reported among other conditions. Since 1982 the PHLS Communicable Diseases Surveillance Centre (CDSC) at Colindale, London, has been monitoring cases of AIDS, using the CDC epidemiological case definition. Confidential reports of patients have been made voluntarily by genito-urinary and other physicians. These have been supported by laboratory reports of opportunistic infections and death certificates (CDSC, 1983). From March 1985 this surveillance has been extended to include patients with positive HTLV-III antibody tests.

STD Services in Other Countries

Eighty per cent of patients with STD are seen by private physicians in the USA, where the clinic service was reduced following the introduction of antibiotics and subsequent decline in cases of syphilis and gonorrhoea. Public health authorities in North America provide state and provincial health departments in large urban areas. These are supplemented by voluntary services.

Dermatovenereology has evolved in many European, Latin American and other countries. This speciality has developed among clinicians previously responsible for the care of patients with skin manifestations of syphilis.

A free and confidential network of specialist STD centres is provided in Australia. Their organisation is similar to that described for the UK.

In conclusion, the comprehensive STD service established over many years in Britain provides a unique framework for managing the broad spectrum of HTLV-III infection.

AIDS – A SEXUALLY TRANSMITTED DISEASE

CDC Case Definition of AIDS

A person (a) with a reliably diagnosed disease that is at least moderately indicative of an underlying cellular immune deficiency – for example, Kaposi's sarcoma in a patient aged less than 60 years, or opportunistic infection; (b) who has no known cause of cellular immune deficiency or any other cause of reduced resistance reported to be associated with the disease.

Causative Agent

Human T cell lymphotropic virus type 3 (HTLV-III).

Incubation Period

15–57 months to date (median 27.5).

Spectrum of HTLV-III Infection

(a) Asymptomatic sero-negative virus-positive persons.
(b) Asymptomatic sero-positive persons.
(c) Persistent generalised lymphadenopathy (PGL).
(d) AIDS-related complex (ARC).
(e) Acquired immune deficiency syndrome (AIDS).

Methods of Transmission of HTLV-III Infection

(a) Sexual transmission.
(b) Spread of blood and blood products.
(c) Accidental exposure.
(d) Transmission from parents to children.
(e) Other routes.

Sexual Transmission of HTLV-III Infection

AIDS, the most severe manifestation of infection with the HTLV-III virus, is considered as part of a clinical spectrum of disease associated with HTLV-III infection and not in isolation. A majority of cases in North America and Europe occur among men who practise receptive or insertive anal coitus with multiple partners. Trauma of the rectal mucosa has been suggested as the portal of viral entry, as occurs in hepatitis B. Therefore, homosexual transmission of HTLV-III infection has been demonstrated.

In the USA sexual transmission has occurred from men, particularly intravenous drug abusers, to their female partners. Sharing of contaminated needles may have contributed to this spread. However, the predominant mode of transmission of AIDS in Central Africa is by heterosexual contact. In Zaire the male-to-female ratio of cases is reported as 1:1.1, which suggests that sexual transmission from women to men may be more common than in western countries (Piot *et al.*, 1984). The importance of this mode of spread in the USA and the UK, and the role of female prostitutes in this transmission, is unknown. Therefore, HTLV-III infection can be considered as a sexually transmitted disease with a similar pattern of transmission to that of hepatitis B.

THE IMPACT OF AIDS ON OTHER SEXUALLY TRANSMITTED DISEASES

A reduction in sexually transmitted diseases acquired by homosexual men in the USA and London (Weller *et al.*, 1984) has been associated with the increased media coverage of AIDS. However, there has been no corresponding decline in rates among heterosexual men.

Increased episodes of STD, in the preceding year, has been considered a risk factor in the development of sero-positivity for HTLV-III, among homosexual men undergoing long-term surveillance (Weber, 1985).

Syphilis

Cases of syphilis have declined in Britain since 1978, owing, in part, to a fall in homosexually acquired disease.

A persistently elevated non-specific serological test (Venereal Disease Research Laboratory test – VDRL) has been demonstrated in some patients with a past history of adequately treated syphilis and concurrent HTLV-III infection. The VDRL antigen reacts with 'reagin', a circulating antibody present in the sera of patients infected with syphilis. The level of 'reagin' is increased as part of the polyclonal hypergammaglobulinaemia found in AIDS-related diseases. Therefore, the VDRL titre remains high.

A gumma of the penile shaft was diagnosed in a patient with PGL. Persistently elevated VDRL titres were recorded despite many documented courses of penicillin for both congenital and acquired syphilis. Immunosuppression is a feature of HTLV-III infection and has been associated with reactivation of avirulent/low-virulence treponemes in lymph nodes, aqueous humour and cerebrospinal fluid. These factors may have contributed to the development of tertiary syphilis in this patient, the gumma healing after high-dose penicillin therapy (Weber, 1985).

There may be difficulty in diagnosing the underlying condition when generalised lymphadenopathy is associated with a high VDRL titre. Retreatment of syphilis is recommended. The potential for HTLV-III infection to reactivate treated treponemal disease is unknown.

Gonorrhoea

Cases of gonorrhoea have declined among homosexual men in London (Weller *et al.*, 1984). Rectal gonorrhoea has decreased, which suggests that patients may be modifying their sexual behaviour in response to the media coverage of AIDS.

Herpes simplex Virus Infection

Prolonged and severe ano-genital herpetic ulceration is associated with ARC and AIDS. Maintenance therapy with oral acyclovir is necessary.

Genital Warts

Condyloma acuminata, unresponsive to conventional therapy are found in

AIDS-related diseases. Wart virus infection has been associated with oral hairy leucoplakia of the tongue, and may be a precursor in the development of squamous cell carcinoma of the tongue and anus. These malignancies have been increasing in incidence in young men in the USA.

Molluscum Contagiosum

Large multiple molluscum situated in the face may be a feature of ARC and AIDS. Treatment is given for cosmetic reasons but may not be effective.

Hepatitis B

The potential for HTLV-III to reactivate hepatitis B infection is unknown. There is no epidemiological evidence to suggest an association between hepatitis B vaccine and AIDS, despite earlier concern (CDC, 1984). At-risk individuals, including male homosexuals, should be offered immunisation (Adler *et al.*, 1983), although the safe sex guidelines protect against the acquisition of this infection.

HTLV-III INFECTION AND DEPARTMENTS OF GENITO-URINARY MEDICINE

General Considerations

Genito-urinary medicine is an out-patient speciality which provides a cost-effective service for the diagnosis, treatment and contact tracing of patients with STD. Clinic premises are often located away from the hospital to which the department is attached. Liaison with other medical colleagues is limited, few patients requiring referral, because of the availability of effective antibiotic therapy. Therefore, genito-urinary medicine has maintained a low profile among other specialities.

Sexual transmission of HTLV-III infection has occurred in the majority of cases. AIDS-related disease may replace syphilis as the STD with the most diverse clinical manifestations. Genito-urinary physicians who wish to manage patients with suspected HTLV-III infection must develop good liaison with their hospital-based colleagues in all specialities.

Our experience of managing patients with AIDS-related disease is based on a large central London department where homosexual men form a high proportion of the clinic load. One-third of all AIDS cases reported in the UK have been seen at St Mary's hospital. A large number of patients with AIDS concern or HTLV-III infection have also been reviewed. The expertise that we have developed cannot be considered typical of that found in all departments of genito-urinary medicine, which vary in size, facilities and clientele.

Routine management of STD, although the responsibility of the individual physician, is similar throughout the country. Guidelines for the out-patient management of concerned patients, at-risk groups and those with proven HTLV-III infection can apply to all departments of genito-urinary medicine. These clinics will be involved in seeing patients with AIDS-related diseases if the recent DHSS guidelines (DHSS, 1985) are followed. Smaller clinics may find it appropriate to liaise with colleagues in general medicine or infectious diseases, at a district level, to provide continuing care and an in-patient facility. Genito-urinary physicians do not have the expertise to deal with the acute medical problems that may develop in AIDS patients. Numbers of at-risk patients may remain too small for specialist clinics to develop, as has occurred within our department.

The Routine Clinic

A clinical examination of at-risk patients, including all homosexual men attending departments of genito-urinary medicine, is necessary at regular intervals (4–6-monthly). PGL can present without symptoms and would not be detected on routine STD screening. This increases the clinic work load, more time being spent on health education and counselling of at-risk groups. An increased awareness of STD, including AIDS, has been caused by recent extensive media coverage and has raised our patients' expectations of the service, contributing to longer waiting times.

An awareness of the range of symptomatology associated with HTLV-III infection is essential (see Chapter 1). Minor symptoms (e.g. malaise and lethargy) cannot be dismissed. Clinical features of HTLV-III infection have already been described (Chapter 1). Specialised investigations have been listed and will not be discussed further.

The minimum number of investigations necessary to establish the diagnosis and assist in clinical management are performed on each patient. This reduces the risk of infection to medical and technical staff. Results must be reviewed by medical personnel so that appropriate action can be taken, where necessary. Good liaison with laboratory staff ensures phoned reports of urgent tests.

Request forms for all investigations should be clearly written. Biohazard labels or flagging must be applied to all forms and specimen containers, stating the risk – e.g. PGL, AIDS. The patient should be informed of the meaning of the biohazard label and why his tests have been flagged.

Disposable equipment (e.g. plastics loops, proctoscopes) should be introduced for use by all patients within the department. Disposable gloves must be used by staff when taking blood from high-risk patients. Vacuum bottles are recommended for all blood tests, eliminating leakage and spillage. Needle-stick injuries are reduced, as resheathing is not necessary. All used needles, syringes and holders should be placed in a secure box prior to disposal. Guidelines for the management of needle-stick injuries for health care workers have been drawn up.

Non-automated laboratory testing of sera is not carried out in high-risk individuals. Therefore, investigations such as serum amylase, paracetamol levels, ESR and monospot testing are not performed in the laboratory.

All specimens from at-risk patients must be bagged and placed separately from those of the routine clinic. They should be stored safely in secure containers, which can be easily sterilised, for early transfer to the laboratory.

Portering staff must be instructed in correct handling techniques for all specimens. This can be arranged by liaison with laboratory technical staff.

Interim safety guidelines have been drawn up (Advisory Committee on Dangerous Pathogens, 1984) and may be modified for use within one's own hospital. These are discussed in Chapters 3 and 6. Regular interdepartmental meetings with laboratory staff are helpful for discussing problems, and provide a good means of liaison.

Patients attending departments of GUM may be concerned individuals, may be sexual contacts of HTLV-III infection or may have AIDS-related diseases. The differential diagnosis should always be considered, as HTLV-III infection is still rare in the UK. For example, secondary syphilis can present as generalised lymphadenopathy but should be excluded before the patient is 'labelled' as PGL.

AIDS patients may present directly to the routine clinic. Hospital admission should be arranged immediately if clinically appropriate – for example, if *Pneumocystis carinii* pneumonia is suspected. Referral may otherwise be arranged to the hospital-based team with overall clinical responsibility for AIDS cases.

The Specialist Clinic

Specialist clinics have been established within our department for patients who are concerned or who are suspected of having HTLV-III infection. These developed when research funding was found to be providing a service commitment, as increased referrals were taken from the routine clinic.

Continuity of care is provided by the same doctor seeing the patient at each visit. A consistent approach in the management of these cases is provided by discussion among those involved in the clinics. Close co-operation is needed with nursing, reception, technical and laboratory staff.

A symptomatic enquiry and physical examination is followed by investigation, as appropriate. These have been discussed in an earlier chapter. A provisional diagnosis is made, the patient being included in one of seven categories (Table 4.1) and informed of the condition. Results are given at follow-up appointment, 7–10 days later, when further information may be given.

The patient may require only reassurance at follow-up before continuing review in the routine clinic. Regular surveillance may be continued in the specialist clinic, although some patients find this too restrictive and wish to continue being seen in the routine clinic.

Sub-specialisation has developed for specific problems, with monthly clinics in dermatology, ophthalmology and ENT. These have been established because of the large numbers of patients seen with AIDS-related diseases who have associated problems. These clinics do not impose on the general patients in these specialities. Increased expertise and research in the management of the raised manifestations of HTLV-III infection can be developed. Overall clinical responsibility remains with the specialist clinic.

Patients with HTLV-III infection or AIDS concern need open access to medical and ancillary health care staff. Sudden deterioration in clinical condition can occur – for example, a rapidly progressive *Pneumocystis carinii* pneumonia, which merits urgent hospital admission and therapy. Relationship problems and attempted suicides may happen as a secondary feature of HTLV-III infection and require staff to be available for counselling.

The number and allocation of hospital beds devoted to AIDS-related disease is a matter of district policy. Access to in-patient beds is necessary for surgical procedures such as lymph node biopsy, which form part of the patient work-up. Beds may be located on one ward and utilised for AIDS cases, minor surgical procedures and other investigations associated with the management of patients with HTLV-III infection. Alternatively, cases may be distributed throughout the hospital, to even out the clinical work on each ward.

Table 4.1 Categories of patients attending departments of GUM with HTLV-III infection

---

(1) The worried well
(2) 'Fear of AIDS'
(3) Sexual partner of an HTLV-III contact, who may be HTLV-III-antibody-positive or -negative
(4) Asymptomatic HTLV-III-positive person
(5) PGL
(6) ARC
(7) AIDS

History

A detailed systematic enquiry, as outlined in this section, is necessary at presentation in all concerned patients and in those with HTLV-III infection: a comprehensive history is essential at follow-up appointments. Sexual practices and other risk factors are sought.

General Health

(a) General health: No symptoms.
Malaise, lethargy or fatigue.
Fever or night sweats.
Enlarged lymph nodes.
Joint pains.

(b) The skin: Non-itchy spots.

Rashes, especially of the face and neck in a person with no prior history of skin disease.

(c) The gastro-intestinal system: Dysphagia.

Colicky abdominal pain.

Loss of weight.

Unexplained diarrhoea.

Peri-anal discomfort and ulceration.

(d) The respiratory system: Unexplained persistent sore throats.

Persistent non-productive cough.

Mild pleuritic chest pain.

Shortness of breath on exertion.

(e) The central nervous system: Headache.

Loss of balance.

Visual loss.

Confusion or fits.

Disturbance of higher centres − e.g. loss of short-term memory; personality changes.

Sexual History

(a) Sexual partner(s): Sexual contact with a partner who has HTLV-III infection. Obtain details and *confirm* accuracy of information.

(b) Sexual practices: Insertive or receptive anal coitus.

(c) Contact history: Number of sexual partners, both known and unknown over the preceding year.

Preferred sexual practices and geographical location of contact.

Other Risk Factors

(a) Intravenous drug usage with sharing of infected equipment.

(b) Haemophilia.

(c) Foreign travel to Haiti, Central Africa or the USA if sexual contact or the sharing of needles or blood transfusion has occurred.

Sexually Transmitted Diseases

Obtain details of any past infection and confirm accuracy of information.

Physical Examination

A physical examination, as outlined in this section, is necessary at each consultation in those patients with HTLV-III infection. The patient should undress to his underpants and be examined in a quiet, well-lit room.

General Considerations

(a) Assess the patient's mental and emotional state.
(b) Note the gait.
(c) Assess the physique for evidence of recent weight loss.

The Mouth

In good light examine the hard palate, fauces, lateral borders and undersurface of the tongue, using a disposable spatula.

The Skin

Note the distribution and morphology of any lesions.

Lymph Nodes

Examine all accessible sites, including the anterior and posterior triangles of the neck, and the supraclavicular, axillary, epitrochlear and inguinal areas.

The Chest

Observe for evidence of central cyanosis or an increased respiratory rate. Full chest examination.

The Abdomen

Exclude hepatic and splenic enlargement; examine for mass.

The Genitalia and the Peri-anal Area

Exclude ulceration; examine for STD.

Optic Fundi

An ophthalmoscopic examination is essential and should be performed in a darkened room.

Patient Management

The Worried Well

History: There may be guilt following an isolated incident such as a casual sexual contact by a heterosexual man with a prostitute or an attempted homosexual experience by a man when drunk. These can be reinforced by media coverage or discussion with friends. No other known risk factors are present.

Physical examination: Normal.

Baseline investigations: None (routine STD screen, if appropriate).

Management: Reassurance. Consider psychological review.
Follow-up: None. Review in routine clinic.

'Fear of AIDS'

History: The patient is 'symptomatic' with a convincing history. No other known
   risk factors are present.
Physical examination: Normal.
Baseline investigations: None (routine STD screen, if appropriate).
Management: Reassurance.
          Need for psychological/psychiatric review.
          These patients should be taken seriously, as some may attempt
          suicide (Weber *et al.*, 1983).

Follow-up: Psychological/psychiatric support is necessary, with the need for
   long-term follow-up. This condition is a new manifestation of
   'venereophobia' and represents an underlying psychiatric disorder —
   in particular, an obsessional personality.

Sexual Partners of HTLV-III Contacts and Asymptomatic HTLV-III Persons

History: A symptomatic enquiry should be performed. Other risk factors should
   be sought.
Physical examination: Normal.
Baseline investigations: Weight.
               Full blood count.
               (HTLV-III antibody if available.)
               (Routine STD screen if appropriate.)
Management: Reassurance.
          Education and counselling.
          Psychological support.
Follow-up: Three-monthly review.
          Recheck history and examination findings.
          Repeat baseline investigations.

PGL, ARC and AIDS

The management of these patients has been adequately covered in Chapter 1.
Sexual contacts should be advised to attend. Reassurance, education, counselling
and psychological support are necessary.

Routine screening for sexually transmitted diseases should be repeated at
regular intervals in patients with HTLV-III infection. Intercurrent STD may
worsen their immune state if not treated promptly.

CONTACT TRACING

Following DHSS recommendations in 1971, health advisers have been established within most departments of genito-urinary medicine to interview patients with syphilis and gonorrhoea about their sexual contacts (Thin, 1984). Information remains within the clinics and is confidential. The decline in cases of gonorrhoea over recent years may be related, in part, to the increased number of personnel working in this field. The role of health advisers has expanded to include health education and counselling in some departments, depending on clinic work load.

Sixty per cent of sexual partners of AIDS patients are sero-positive for HTLV-III infection. Contact-tracing of these patients with counselling, advice on sexual practices and health education may be of value in limiting the spread of HTLV-III infection. This may only become apparent when a satisfactory treatment is available. The health advisers within the clinics, certainly those in London, would have difficulty taking on the task of contact-tracing AIDS patients, because of their existing work load. Should contact-tracing be applied to all patients with HTLV-III infection, it would be impossible to achieve with existing manpower.

SCREENING FOR HTLV-III INFECTION

Screening for the presence of HTLV-III antibody in at-risk populations, with education and counselling of those found to be positive, is the only available method of confining this infection. Compulsory screening of blood donors has been introduced in the UK to prevent transmission by transfusion or blood products.

Which test?   Several American tests for HTLV-III antibody are available. A British one is awaited. The reliability of the test is important and may reflect the expertise of the laboratory. In low-risk groups, such as blood donors or patients attending some provincial departments of genito-urinary medicine, it is essential to have a low false-positive rate.

Which patients?   Recent publicity in the gay press and interested organisations has either recommended that the individual should be free to make up his own mind on the need for testing or actively advised against it. Advice has been given to all, whether at risk or not, to modify their life-style and practice safer sex. The patient should be informed that the HTLV-III antibody test is available. The wishes of the individual should be respected, except, perhaps, prior to major general surgery, where being sero-positive may affect patient management.

A positive result   The patient must be informed of the result. A positive test indicates prior infection with HTLV-III virus and the potential for transmitting the infection. It does not mean that the individual has AIDS. Over a 2 year period, about 10% of patients who are HTLV-III-positive may develop AIDS, another 35% may have PGL or ARC and the remaining 50% will be healthy. The long-term prognosis is unknown. Counselling services are necessary, to advise and educate the person on the interpretation of the result. Long-term support and follow-up may be required.

A negative result   The patient must be informed of the result and counselling on modification in life-style to prevent the acquisition of the disease. Annual screening is advised, to detect later sero-conversion. The patient may be infectious for the HTLV-III virus although antibody-negative. A screening programme should not be introduced unless the consequences can be dealt with.

COUNSELLING

All patients with HTLV-III infection should be informed of the clinical diagnosis and the results of antibody screening. The implications of this should be discussed. Adequate diet and exercise is recommended. Social contact by others with AIDS-related diseases is not a risk factor. Safe sex guidelines are being recommended for all homosexual men, unless in well-established regular relationships, although difficult for some to accept. Efficacy of condoms has not been established, but they may reduce transmission of the HTLV-III virus. Simple hygiene — for example, personal use of razors, toothbrushes, etc. — is essential. Equipment used for piercing the skin for tattoos, acupuncture, etc., either should not be utilised or should be sterilised after each usage. Blood and body organs should not be offered for donation.

Counselling may be carried out by any interested member of the clinic team, provided that there is consistency of information, sufficient time and reinforcement at subsequent visits. With the introduction of HTLV-III antibody screening, larger numbers of patients will require this service. Group meetings may develop for these persons, or they may wish to attend voluntary organisations to gain more information.

CONFIDENTIALITY

The success of the STD service in the UK, demonstrated by a low rate of infection per head of population when compared with other Western countries, is based on the patient's knowledge that all confidential information remains within the clinic. Medical secrecy is protected by statute. Certain details may be disclosed to doctors or health advisers, to facilitate contact-tracing and treatment of STD. The case notes are stored within the clinic, separate from the hospital records, and are not allowed to leave the department. Clinic staff are trained in confidentiality (Catterall, 1980).

A patient who is HTLV-III-antibody-positive is advised to notify his general practitioner and his dentist. Problems can arise in confidentiality if the patient's homosexuality is unknown to them. Medical records are less secure in these situations. The result may be included in medical reports for employers and insurance companies, to the detriment of the patient, who may be otherwise well. Some gay organisations advise the use of false names within the clinic, to preserve confidentiality.

The HTLV-III status of patients referred to hospital may be required, especially if surgery is contemplated (Glazer and Dudley, 1985). Concern about confidentiality may stop some patients from disclosing this information or prevent them from being screened, which places medical and ancillary staff at risk if inappropriate precautions are taken.

HTLV-III infection is notified in a confidential and voluntary manner to the DHSS for identification purposes. Statutory notification was considered but turned down after informed debate. Compulsory notification of STD was attempted during World War II. This was a total failure, because physicians objected to the loss of their patient's confidentiality. A physician's responsibility in GUM is to the individual patient. Compulsory powers have been introduced for the patient who is a health risk to himself and others, but who refuses hospital admission.

Adequate counselling of the patient, health care workers and the general public may reduce the stigma attached to the HTLV-III virus. Improved theatre and laboratory facilities will mean that all cases can be treated in a safe manner as at-risk specimens.

CONCLUSIONS

More than three-quarters of all AIDS cases have been seen among several large teaching hospitals in the four Thames regions. They have developed into 'centres of excellence' and have an obligation to provide a teaching and research commitment. Training courses are necessary for health care workers to gain basic expertise in the management of HTLV-III infection.

The predicted new patient case load for 1985 is 400 AIDS cases and 2000 persons with PGL. All teaching hospitals and many district general hospitals will become involved in care. The cost of managing AIDS and HTLV-III infection is considerable and should be evenly distributed.

Provincial departments of GUM will have neither the facilities nor the work load to develop a specialised service. However, they will become involved in the management of HTLV-III infection over the coming years, with increasing numbers of affected persons. Liaison with medical colleagues will provide integrated out-patient care of such patients. The hospital-based specialist will take over the acute problems and in-patient management.

AIDS and HTLV-III infection have brought the speciality of genito-urinary medicine into public focus. The clinical spectrum of the AIDS-related diseases is a tremendous health challenge. The integrated system of clinics within the UK provides the basic structure for concentrating expertise and containing the spread of HTLV-III infection. 'However, if proper planning and adequate resources are not forthcoming for genito-urinary medicine then the speciality cannot be expected to assume responsibility for containment of HTLV-III infection with its ever-present risk to the heterosexual community.' (Evans *et al.*, 1985)

REFERENCES

Adler, M. W., Belsey, E. M., McCutchan, J. A. and Mindel, A. (1983). *Br. Med. J.*, **286**, 1621

Advisory Committee on Dangerous Pathogens (1984). *Acquired Immune Deficiency Syndrome (AIDS) – Interim Guidelines*. DHSS, London

Anon. (1985). Sexually transmitted diseases: Extract from the Annual Report of the Chief Medical Officer of the Department of Health and Social Security for the year 1983. *Genitourin. Med.*, **61**, 204

Catterall, R. D. (1980). *Br. J. Vener. Dis.*, **56**, 263

Catterall, R. D. (1984). *Br. J. Vener. Dis.*, **60**, 337

CDC (1984). *Morbidity and Mortality Weekly Report*, **33**, 685

CDSC (1983). *Br. Med. J.*, **287**, 407

Department of Health and Social Security (1985). *Acquired Immune Deficiency Syndrome (AIDS) – General Information for Doctors*. DHSS, London

Dubois, R. M., Branthwaite, M. A., Mikhail, J. R. and Botten, J. G. (1981). *Lancet*, **ii**, 1339

Evans, B. A., Lawrence, A., Oates, J. K. and Samarasinghe, P. L. (1985). *Lancet*, **i**, 1338

Glazer, G. and Dudley, H. (1985). *Br. Med. J.*, **290**, 852

Green, J. and Miller, D. (1985). *Br. J. Hosp. Med.*, **33**, 353

Mortimer, P. P., Jesson, W. J., Vandervelde, E. M. and Pereira, M. S. (1985). *Br. Med. J.*, **290**, 1176

Piot, P., Quinn, T. C., Taelman, H. *et al.* (1984). *Lancet*, **ii**, 65

Thin, R. N. (1984). *Br. J. Vener. Dis.*, **60**, 269

Weber, J. (1985). Personal communication

Weber, J. and Goldmeier, D. (1983). *Br. Med. J.*, **287**, 420

Weller, I. V. D., Hindley, D. J., Adler, M. W. and Meldrum, J. T. (1984). *Br. Med. J.*, **289**, 1041

5

AIDS-related Problems in the Management of Haemophilia

Peter B.A. Kernoff and Riva R. Miller

Haemophilia is a rare disease, with a world-wide prevalence of about 100 per million of the population. Without treatment, it causes crippling from an early age, and premature death. It can have devastating effects on family and social relationships, and on opportunities and ability to fully integrate into society. Modern therapy with blood products has been dramatically successful in preventing and alleviating the worst effects of the disease. Before AIDS, the prospects of a normal life had to many never seemed brighter, a mood of optimism which was fuelled not only by the expectations and hopes of patients themselves, but also by health care professionals and commercial interests. In the words of a 40-year-old man with severe haemophilia: 'With successful treatment for bleeding, I thought most of the battle was won. With AIDS, it's starting all over again.'

BLEEDING IN HAEMOPHILIA

There are two types of haemophilia, A and B, which are identical in their clinical manifestations and modes of inheritance. In haemophilia A, the commoner variety, bleeding is caused by a deficiency of an essential protein in the blood, factor VIII, which is needed for normal blood coagulation. In haemophilia B (Christmas Disease) factor IX is deficient. Both disorders are inherited as X-linked recessive traits. With rare exceptions, haemophilia is confined to males.

The clinical severity of haemophilia correlates with the level of factor VIII/IX in circulating blood. Patients with severe disease (<2 u/dl factor VIII/IX) suffer from repeated, spontaneous and painful bleeding into muscles and joints, which, if untreated, rapidly leads to irreversible damage. Only 20 years ago, such events would require long periods of painful immobilisation in bed, perhaps in hospital, and analgesic dependence was common. Now most bleeding episodes can be rapidly aborted by the prompt administration of clotting factor concentrates, often given at home or at work. Although modern therapy has had a profoundly beneficial impact on haemophilia, bleeding still remains a dominant problem for most patients, and the most common cause of death.

PLASMA PRODUCT THERAPY: DILEMMAS OF TREATMENT

Both factor VIII and factor IX are constituents of normal plasma, which must be frozen within a few hours of collection for it to be useful for therapeutic purposes. Fresh frozen plasma (FFP) remained in routine use for the treatment of haemophiliacs in the UK until the early 1970s, when it was superseded by different types of clotting factor concentrates.

An early concentrate, cryoprecipitate, accounts for about 5% of factor VIII usage in the UK. It has the particular advantages of simplicity of manufacture and only low donor exposure for patients. The potential advantage of low donor pool size may be lost in patients with severe haemophilia, who usually need frequent transfusions. In most Western countries, chemically fractionated, lyophilised, clotting factor concentrates are now preferred for the routine treatment of severe haemophilia. These products are produced on an industrial scale, usually from plasma pools to which 1500-10 000 donors have contributed. They are stable, can be stored in a domestic refrigerator, and are of designated potency, thus allowing dosing according to normal pharmacological principles.

A majority of haemophiliacs are managed on 'demand' regimens — i.e. an intravenous infusion of clotting factor is given as soon as possible after bleeding becomes apparent, with the objective of temporarily raising the patient's plasma factor VIII/IX level. After infusion, levels of factor VIII and IX fall away rapidly. Hence, frequent treatment is often needed to maintain plasma levels high enough to control major bleeding. Since the introduction of factor VIII and IX concentrates for routine therapy in the early 1970s, attitudes towards the use of plasma products have changed markedly. Factor VIII and IX concentrates are no longer regarded as special preparations, for use only in emergencies. Rather, they are viewed as essential drugs, to be used liberally and with the overall objective of allowing as normal a life as possible. Self-administration ('home treatment') regimens have allowed patients to achieve a high degree of independence from hospitals, and to embark on activities which would have been unthinkable for haemophiliacs even a decade ago.

Since the recognition of AIDS as a risk of blood product therapy, we have noticed only a small reduction in concentrate used by severely affected patients. For most, the benefits of therapy remain paramount: 'I'm treating myself the same — if I get it, I get it. I fear the isolation and dependency that results from being unable to walk, and I can't face the agonies of pain again.'

For parents of young children, the dilemmas of treatment can be more intense. They see older, crippled patients, and know that concentrate therapy is the only way of avoiding long-term complications. Often, knowing that the mother was a carrier of haemophilia, they took a decision to have children because treatment seemed so effective. The mother of a 5-year-old child said: 'I know that the infusion I'm giving him may make him die, but I must treat him. I hate it.' These burdens of increased responsibility and stress are shared by the parents of older children, and there has been a re-emergence of patterns of over-protective behaviour that were common before effective treatment became available. A 15-year-old boy reported: 'I don't treat my bleeds so quickly. Dad says I've got to cut down. He's told my brother not to risk bleeds by running over rough ground.'

PLASMA PRODUCT SUPPLY

A long-standing problem in haemophilia care has been to obtain sufficient quantities of therapeutic plasma products. Because of the relatively small number of patients with haemophilia B, this has been less of a problem with factor IX than with factor VIII. Over the last 15 years, the amount of factor VIII used in the UK has increased at a rate of about 20% annually. The reasons are clear: *demand* has increased because the benefits of more intensive treatment have been obvious; *supply* of factor VIII has been available both to meet and to fuel this demand.

In production of factor VIII, as with several other plasma products, the UK is not self-sufficient. To meet demand, the supply of home-produced material has had to be augmented since the early 1970s by importation of increasingly large quantities of commercially produced factor VIII concentrates, mainly from the USA. Currently about two-thirds of all factor VIII used in the UK is imported. At least until recently, all factor IX used has been produced by the National Health Service (NHS).

In the USA, which probably produces at least 75% of total world supplies, plasma products are made by commercial companies from plasma collected on a massive scale from paid donors, and both plasma and finished products are regarded as commodities in which there is an international trade and brokerage system, and the prices and availability of which are determined by market forces. Although it is difficult to establish with certainty, products now imported into the UK are probably derived from plasma collected in the continental USA. In past years, plasma collected in other countries, including developing nations, was probably used to make the finished products which were distributed both within and outside the USA. Of relevance to AIDS and its transmission is the fact that commercial plasma collection facilities were established in several central African countries.

The possibility that reliance on imported plasma products might carry increased risks of transmissible disease has been appreciated for many years. A long-standing and still unresolved problem is post-infusion hepatitis, especially that due to non-A, non-B (NANB) agents. A large proportion of regularly treated haemophiliacs have sustained abnormalities of biochemical liver function tests, and many have biopsy-proven chronic liver disease. Most haemophiliacs are aware of the risks of hepatitis which accompany the use of clotting factor concentrates, although they may not appreciate their magnitude. The benefits of therapy are usually perceived to outweigh the risks, perhaps especially because the evolution of chronic liver disease, unlike that of AIDS, takes place over decades rather than a few years.

It has long been accepted in the UK that it would be desirable to achieve self-sufficiency in blood products. Unfortunately, acceptance of the principle has not led to realisation in practice. A recent advance has been investment in a new NHS plasma fractionation factory at Elstree, Hertfordshire, UK. It remains to be seen whether sufficient quantities of plasma can be collected to enable this plant to operate at full capacity. History provides few reasons for optimism:

'Blood voluntarily and freely given by the healthy to those in need is a manifestation of the values we should all strive to maintain in a society.' (Dr David Owen, UK Minister of Health, 1976)

'Self-sufficiency expected by mid 1977.' (DHSS Press Release)

'A disgrace to be included in a fourth world . . . an indictment of what happens in a socialised system.' (President of Alpha Therapeutics Inc., on the UK blood supply system)

Relatives of haemophiliacs have traditionally been motivated blood donors, particularly because of the long-standing plasma supply problem in the UK. For some, donation has assuaged feelings of guilt. The exclusion of sexual partners of haemophiliacs from blood donation has underlined the infective aspects of the condition, and that the complications of the disease are not confinable to patients. Possibilities of social isolation and ostracisation consequent on labelling as 'contaminated', so common for haemophiliacs in the pretreatment era, have been reawakened. Increasingly, the focus of blame has shifted from commercial companies. The wife of a 54-year-old haemophiliac commented: 'Maybe AIDS is new, but they were talking about hepatitis 10 years ago. If the Americans can make enough factor VIII to export, why can't we make enough for ourselves? We wouldn't have this problem if the Government had kept its promises and done something. It's too late now.'

HEALTH CARE DELIVERY: HAEMOPHILIA CENTRES

The concept of centralising treatment at special Haemophilia Centres originated in the UK in the early 1950s. Initially, the main function of the Centres was diagnosis. As effective treatment became available, activities expanded and responsibility for organisation was taken over by the Department of Health Now a national network of Centres provides comprehensive care for patients with haemophilia and related disorders.

The statutory functions of the largest Haemophilia Centres (Reference Centres) are wide-ranging. They include provision of primary and specialised clinical care; specialist laboratory facilities; educational and research commitments; responsibilities for the co-ordination of community services and blood product supply; collection of statistics; financial planning; and genetic and psychosocial counselling. This well-developed organisational infrastructure is certainly better placed to respond to AIDS-related problems than are the services available to most patients in other high-risk groups.

With the increasing availability of plasma products, management has become predominantly out-patient-based, with a large proportion of severely affected patients being maintained on 'home treatment' regimens. This has brought patients independence, but also problems of personal responsibility and choice. A difficulty for Centres has sometimes been to maintain contact with patients, in order to identify and contain emerging problems. This has been achieved by establishing formalised multidisciplinary review clinics, which patients attend at 6- or 12-monthly intervals. These clinics, together with existing facilities for counselling, have proved a useful opportunity to deal with and anticipate AIDS-related problems.

Because haemophilia is a life-long disease, patients may spend many years, even a lifetime, under the care of one Centre. They establish close relationships with staff, and not infrequently the boundaries between personal and professional relationships become blurred. This can cause problems when difficult and multifaceted issues such as AIDS have to be dealt with, since they may necessitate intrusion into a patient's private life to a degree to which staff are unaccustomed. For example, one young staff nurse who shares responsibility for informing patients about possible risk prevention had difficulty advising men of her own age about the use of condoms. A particular problem for staff is dealing with the uncertainties of AIDS. Reassurances which patients seek cannot often be provided. Their anxieties can be expressed as anger, often directed against the Centre and its staff. It is important to create opportunities for staff to meet to discuss these issues. Staff need to maintain professional boundaries in order to provide the patients and their families with the support which they seek.

HAEMOPHILIA SOCIETIES AND THE WORLD FEDERATION OF HEMOPHILIA

The development of haemophilia care in the UK has by no means been solely dependent on the efforts of professionals. Haemophiliacs, and their relatives, friends and sympathisers, have contributed to a major extent, especially through the activities of the Haemophilia Society, founded in the early 1940s. The Society is a powerful pressure group and has a major commitment to fundraising. Most recently it has been active in disseminating information and advice on AIDS-related issues. Following the foundation of the Haemophilia Society in the UK, many other countries established their own national organisations. This led in 1963 to the formation of the World Federation of Hemophilia (WFH). The WFH has established a 'World Hemophilia AIDS Center' in Los Angeles, which has functions in international surveillance and information exchange.

ANTI-HTLV-III SEROLOGY: 'THE TEST'

Considering the number of patients in the UK who, for many years, have been massively exposed to clotting factor concentrates, the number of haemophiliacs known to have had full-blown AIDS is small. Although under-reporting is possible, only 8 patients, among some 2500 treated annually, are known to have developed the syndrome. None of these has been under our care.

In a sero-epidemiological study carried out in late 1984 in a population of 226 haemophiliacs attending our Centre, anti-HTLV-III was detected only in patients who had been exposed to commercial factor VIII concentrates in the previous 6 years. In this group the positivity rate was 94/132 (71%). Patients who had been treated with NHS-derived products alone during this period – i.e. with cryoprecipitate and/or factor VIII/IX concentrates – were all sero-negative. However, two of these patients (one treated with NHS factor VIII and one with NHS factor IX) sero-converted in 1985. Clearly, at least until recently, only imported concentrates were associated with a risk of HTLV-III transmission. The highest sero-positivity rate (86%) was found in patients treated with commercial factor VIII in 1984. Retrospective examination of stored serum samples obtained from a cohort of intensively treated patients sero-positive for anti-HTLV-III in 1984 showed that 40% had sero-converted in 1980, positive results first occurring in 1979. In early 1985, 14 of the total 96 sero-positive patients had, or had had, unexplained lymphadenopathy, in one case associated with herpes zoster infection. None had AIDS. Thus, sero-positivity for anti-HTLV-III in our patients is about seven times more common than unexplained lymphadenopathy and, by extrapolation, probably about 100 times more common than full-blown AIDS.

Because of the uncertainties of interpretation, we have not viewed the anti-HTLV-III test as being useful in management, and recommendations made to patients have, in general, not differed according to their serological status. In the carrying out of serological studies, patients who have wanted to know the test result – virtually all – have been told. Despite very full explanations of the problems of interpretation, most view a positive result as being indicative of a risk of AIDS and probable infectivity. The latter conclusion is reinforced by hospital regulations which stratify risk according to serological status. Knowledge of a positive result often causes considerable anxiety, which can adversely affect work, concentration and personal relationships. One young man said: 'I can't get it out of my head that I'm positive. It's quite awful.'

A negative result is often taken to mean freedom from risk. A 30-year-old man, after hearing the result of his test, told his friends, who included several other haemophiliacs, that he was 'clear'. Three months later he was found to have sero-converted.

PREVENTION OF HTLV-III TRANSMISSION BY IV THERAPY: STERILISATION OF CONCENTRATES

As has already been discussed, the fact that clotting factor concentrates could be contaminated with hepatitis viruses, especially NANB agents, was recognised well before the appearance of AIDS. Growing concerns about liver disease in the late 1970s induced major fractionators to invest heavily in the production of 'reduced-risk' products. Heat-treated commercial factor VIII became available for clinical trial in the UK in the early 1980s, and the results for the initial studies started to become known in 1984. They were disappointing. At best, the incidence of post-infusion NANB hepatitis was only marginally reduced. Ironically, just at the time the results of these trials became known, evidence became available that the processes which had failed to eliminate NANB agents were effective against HTLV-III. Thus, the new products found an immediate market, despite their imperfections. Not only this, but they were used in preference to NHS factor VIII, which, for logistic reasons, could only be made available in a heated version in very small quantities. Now virtually all factor VIII concentrate used in the UK is heat-treated. Because of continuing NHS supply problems, however, dependence on imported commercial products is, if anything, greater than it previously was.

For patients with haemophilia B treated with NHS factor IX concentrate, and those with mild disease who are not normally treated with concentrates, resolution of the product infectivity problem has not been so straightforward. Probably because of its different method of preparation, factor IX concentrate seems less likely than factor VIII to carry a risk of HTLV-III transmission. Also, as a UK-derived product, less contamination would be expected. There are some concerns that heating may cause an increased risk of thrombogenicity. At the time of writing, logistic problems have prevented heat 'sterilisation' of factor IX concentrate by the NHS. Therefore, physicians have had to make a decision as to whether to change to heat-treated commercial products, which may carry increased risks other than HTLV-III transmission, or to continue using standard NHS factor IX. In a climate of differing opinions, we have chosen the former course.

To reduce risks of transmitting hepatitis, it has been our policy for several years to avoid treating patients with mild haemophilia with concentrates. Sometimes pharmacological intervention is sufficient; otherwise, plasma or cryoprecipitate is used. Although these products cannot be sterilised, the risk of HTLV-III transmission is considered remote, especially since donor screening has become more stringent. However, heat-treated concentrates may be preferred for some patients. In the longer term, the availability of 'synthetic' bioengineered therapeutic products will eliminate all risks of viral transmission. Whether this prospect will inhibit development of safer versions of current materials remains to be seen.

HAVING CHILDREN

With the primary objective of preventing haemophilia, a great deal of effort has been expended on developing techniques for detection of the carrier state and antenatal diagnosis. Available methods are now sophisticated, and genetic counselling is an important component of a haemophilia care service. The over-all impact of these techniques on the birth rate of haemophiliacs has, as yet, been minimal. One reason is the view, especially among parents of young children, that haemophilia is no longer a serious disease, and that blood product therapy can 'make life normal'.

For many couples wanting children, AIDS has changed this perception. Not only is there the possibility of a haemophilic child contracting AIDS from his treatment, but also a father with haemophilia might, through his wife, infect his unborn child. A 35-year-old man with haemophilia said: 'I'd decided to take my chances with treatment, but we couldn't risk a child getting AIDS. I know we're both getting older, but we can't have children at the moment.'

PERSONAL AND SEXUAL RELATIONSHIPS: 'LABELLING'

A long-standing problem for haemophiliacs, especially when they reach their teens, is how they should define themselves to others. Common dilemmas are to decide whether, when and how to tell others about their disease. Many patients avoid telling sexual partners until late in the development of their relationships — rejection is common and the fear and anticipation of this happening can cause stress and anxiety. Many haemophiliacs, more so in the past, avoid telling employers, colleagues at work and social contacts. A related problem, that of being labelled as handicapped or 'different', often starts in school, and adds to feelings of isolation. Some patients react by dismissing and rejecting their haemophilia, taking up pursuits and occupations which may jeopardise their physical health, but can compensate for feelings of being 'less than a man'. A young motorbike messenger with haemophilia said: 'I refuse to let haemophilia affect my life and keep away from the Centre as much as possible. Coming to the Centre reminds me I have haemophilia. My boss doesn't know I have it. He'd probably sack me if he did.'

For obvious reasons, AIDS has added enormously to these burdens, and in-creased clinical surveillance has made such attitudes difficult to sustain. Long-standing fears that others could 'catch' a haemophiliacs' disease have become a reality. The uncertainties of developing AIDS or carrying infection have added new dimensions to the dilemmas of coping with the bleeding disease. Labelling has become linked with homosexuals and drug addicts. Patients and their parents report:

'My wife's off me, she won't even kiss me.'

'My wife's pregnant, I've told her I'm off sex.'

'I've stopped going to the pub. They'll think I can pass it on through my glass.'

'It's hard enough. I don't want my son linked to those others. I lie awake wondering how he'll get a job if they know he has haemophilia.'

'A parent of a child at my son's school phoned. She said I should keep him out of school.'

DEALING WITH THE PROBLEMS: COUNSELLING

In attempting to deal with the problems caused by AIDS-related issues, we feel it is important to appreciate at the outset that in the present climate of uncertainties, it will never be possible to completely allay anxiety. What can be attempted, in addition to providing information and making specific recommendations on practical issues, is to help people cope with and contain their anxieties. Most commonly, this can be accomplished by structured discussion, which helps to lessen stress and demote AIDS from a concern of frightening and overwhelming proportions to one which has defined limits and can be ranked among the many other problems with which individuals and families have to cope.

Experience gained from our existing system of comprehensive care has helped us to deal with AIDS-related problems, but these have still imposed great strains on resources, particularly of time and manpower. Although information on AIDS has been available from a large number of sources, most patients have looked to their Centre for advice and help. Staff availability is important. Some centres have disseminated information by holding 'mass meetings'. We have thought an individual or family approach to be more likely to be helpful, although logistically more difficult. In particular, we have used 6-monthly review clinics to assess degrees of knowledge and concern about AIDS-related issues. Family members are encouraged to attend at the same time as patients. These clinics are followed up, as necessary, by additional and more detailed counselling sessions, which provide continued support. Group meetings have also been useful not only to share information, but also in helping participants define, cope with and anticipate problems.

In discussing AIDS-related issues with patients, their families and staff, we think that certain general principles are important:

- Take nothing for granted. Despite the publicity given to AIDS, many patients have misconceptions. Some may be very concerned, but others may not.

- Check what people know in stages, before giving or correcting information.
- Be matter-of-fact and interested, and don't appear emotional or alarmed.
- Reflect on their last sentence, and use this for the next question rather than moving on to a new topic. This helps to ensure that you move at their level of comprehension.
- Use questions to keep people to the point, help them define and quantify problems, and seek their own solutions.
- If they become stressed, angry or confused, offer another appointment. This helps them to feel less lost and their problems more contained. Follow-up appointments are normally offered at not less than a month, to allow time for interactions triggered by interviews to take effect.

Some specific examples will be given of questions and responses which might be used in counselling sessions. Initial objectives are to assess the level of concern about AIDS, extent of knowledge, and whether help is being sought:

'If I was to ask you what your major concern was today, what would it be?'
'Where does AIDS rank with all your other concerns?'
'What do you understand about AIDS?'
'How do you think you and your contacts might get AIDS?'

Many people have difficulty in answering this last question without encouragement. Some patients have not discussed the matter with their wives or girl friends, hoping to protect their partners from anxiety, and being afraid of the consequences for themselves. Clearly, this causes tensions in relationships and increased burdens for the patient. To help them think more constructively, and share their fears, one could ask:

'If your wife were here, what do you think she would say?'
'What would be her greatest concern? Would she be worried more for you or for herself?'
'How do you think you could approach sex differently, and still achieve an acceptable level of satisfaction?'

The main threat of AIDS is to personal relationships. It is important to know how much patients are talking to others, and to whom, to be able to gauge how they are dealing with their uncertainties:

'Who else have you spoken to about AIDS?'
'Who has spoken to you about AIDS? What did they say?'
'Are people treating you differently? Who? In what way?

Often, answering questions with questions rather than information or explanations can help people think in a more focused way, set limits on their anxieties and identify ways of dealing with them. In answering the questions 'How will I know if I've got AIDS?', 'How will I cope?' or 'How can I stop thinking about it all the time?' one could respond:

'What do you know about the symptoms?'
'If you thought you had it, who would you turn to first?'
'How much is all the time? All day and night? Two hours a day?'

Group meetings, attended by both patients and staff, can supplement individual or family counselling by providing opportunities for participants to share experiences and concerns, and explore ways of dealing with their problems. They are most useful when planned and led by a professional with expertise in the field. As in individual counselling, issues can be raised which, because they have not previously been considered, can cause additional worries. The mutually supportive relationships which develop in groups are helpful in coping with these.

SOME CONCLUSIONS

Haemophiliacs and their families are not unfamiliar with many of the anxieties and dilemmas of AIDS, but they had hoped that they belonged to the past. Major scientific advances which have occurred in the last 2 years have brought the possibilities of safe therapy, or even a cure for haemophilia, very close. Unfortunately, these advances have come too late to have much impact on AIDS-related problems. Tragically, for haemophiliacs in the UK, these problems could largely have been avoided if effective action had been taken to achieve self-sufficiency in blood products. Both figuratively and literally, the price is now being paid.

6
Nursing

Elizabeth Jenner, Anthony Levi and David Houghton

GENERAL INFORMATION

Acquired Immune Deficiency Syndrome (AIDS) is caused by a human T cell lymphotropic virus (HTLV-III). It has an incubation period of from 6 months to at least 5 years depending on the risk group.

Those persons at risk of acquiring the virus are male homosexuals, intravenous drug abusers who share contaminated needles and syringes, and haemophiliacs and others who have received contaminated blood products. There have also been some cases in heterosexual partners of individuals in the above groups and in infants born to mothers in whom infection is likely.

The virus is spread by sexual intercourse and blood.

Patients with AIDS suffer from Kaposi's sarcoma and/or opportunistic infections such as *Pneumocystis carinii* pneumonia (PCP).

PART 1: INFECTION CONTROL ASPECTS OF CARE

FOREWORD

In accordance with the Interim Guidelines on Acquired Immune Deficiency Syndrome (AIDS) prepared by the Advisory Committee on Dangerous Pathogens (1984), the Infection Control Team at St Mary's Hospital, London W2, has written AIDS/HTLV-III policies for care in the community, wards and specialist departments (e.g. X-ray, theatre) and procedures for specific activities (e.g. specimen handling, and care and removal of infected bodies).

Local documents should be read, understood and adhered to by all relevant staff. The Infection Control Nurse and Infection Control Officer are always available for advice and consultation. This contribution is based on the St Mary's policies and procedures, which have been implemented throughout Paddington and North Kensington Health Authority.

INTRODUCTION

Caring for a patient with AIDS or an AIDS-related disease poses an unusual challenge from the infection control perspective. The patient is a potential source of infection and at the same time is at great risk of acquiring infections with opportunistic pathogens.

INFECTION CONTROL PRECAUTIONS

Infection control precautions should be directed towards: (a) preventing blood-to-blood spread of HTLV-III; (b) protecting the patient from further infections. Therefore, the principles of source isolation and protective isolation have to be applied concurrently.

Source Isolation

The patient who is HTLV-III-antibody-positive is capable of spreading the virus through blood and semen. Additionally, he may be infected with other organisms, such as cytomegalovirus, *Salmonella* spp. or *Mycobacterium tuberculosis*. In order to limit the spread of these organisms, infection control measures are designed to prevent cross-infection.

Protective Isolation

The patient is susceptible to opportunistic infections because of his immune deficiency. Therefore, infection control measures are designed to protect him from both endogenous and exogenous sources of infection.

For these reasons the patient is ideally nursed in a single room. This also gives him privacy and a quiet atmosphere. He can talk freely to visitors and health care workers without the fear of confidential information being overheard.

If the patient is suffering from profuse and frequent diarrhoea, he is considerably less embarrassed and inconvenienced in a single room than if he is cared for in an open ward.

A quiet atmosphere is essential for the care of those suffering from a disturbance of the central nervous system, such as meningitis.

The main disadvantage of a single room is that it can create a feeling of *isolation*. The patient may feel 'cut off' physically, socially and psychologically. Staff must therefore be acutely aware of this and modify their care accordingly. If the patient is well enough, he may welcome the provision of entertainment such as television, radio and library books. The support of friends and relatives can be encouraged by flexible visiting hours and access to a mobile telephone.

A patient in a single room is not as easily observed as a patient in the open ward. Furthermore, a patient with AIDS frequently requires high-dependency and intensive nursing care. Staffing levels may need to be increased to meet these demands.

Inadequate staffing levels jeopardise the health and safety not only of the patient, but also of the staff themselves. An increase in stress, both physical and psychological, can quickly lead to a lowering of staff morale. When such a situation exists, infection control measures are likely to be compromised.

BASIC NURSING CARE

An ill AIDS patient may be suffering from a variety of symptoms, such as a dry unproductive cough, fever, anorexia, nausea and vomiting, profuse diarrhoea and profound weight loss. He is likely to be anxious, tired and irritable. He is at risk of infection not only because he is immunocompromised, but also because of the sequelae that develop if his symptoms go unchecked. These include undernourishment, dehydration, electrolyte imbalance and a high stress level. The nurse who cares for this patient requires a sound knowledge of the behavioural and life sciences, and will use all his or her basic nursing skills.

Problems require prompt identification, swift intervention and critical evaluation of the outcome.

Nutrition

The patient's nutritional status is an extremely important aspect of his care. He may be encouraged to eat and drink if food and beverages that he actually likes are presented in an attractive manner. Small meals served as often as 2-hourly may be preferred if the patient has gastro-intestinal problems.

The patient's diet may need to be modified in some way, such as an increase in carbohydrates and protein and a decrease in fats. He may not be able to tolerate feeding via the gastro-intestinal tract, in which case total parenteral nutrition will be instituted. In any event, the dietician should be consulted.

Elimination

The HTLV-III virus has not been isolated from urine or faeces. The patient should be enabled to micturate and defaecate normally.

If he is continent, he can eliminate directly into the toilet in his room. In the absence of such private facilities, a commode or urinal should be provided and emptied immediately after use (see page 101).

Diarrhoea may result in faecal incontinence and cause the patient severe embarrassment. Soiled incontinence pads should be discarded as per infected waste (see page 101). An infective cause should be sought by the prompt collection of specimens for microbiological investigation. Cytomegalovirus, bacteria such as *Salmonella* spp. or enteric protozoal pathogens such as *Giardia lamblia*,

Entamoeba histolytica and *Cryptosporidium* may be found. The efficacy of anti-diarrhoeal agents that may have been prescribed should be assessed and reported to the doctor.

Urinary incontinence should preferably be managed by the use of externally fitted appliances such as condoms. Invasive devices such as indwelling bladder catheters put the patient at great risk not only of urinary tract infection, but also of Gram-negative septicaemia.

The patient should be reminded of the importance of hand washing after elimination and before eating.

Respiration

About half of all AIDS patients develop pneumonia caused by the protozoan *Pneumocystis carinii* (Communicable Disease Report 84/52). This opportunistic pathogen is the single most common cause of death in these patients. Symptoms include dyspnoea, tachypnoea and a dry unproductive cough. Blood gas levels may require correction. In severe cases the patient may need assisted ventilation. Chest X-rays are taken and fibre-optic bronchoscopy is usually performed to aid diagnosis. Bronchial washings are obtained for microscopy and culture, and a lung biopsy for cytology.

Bacterial causes of chest infections include *Haemophilus influenzae, Mycobacterium tuberculosis*, atypical mycobacteria such as *Mycobacterium avium-intracellulare* and *Legionella pneumophila*, the bacterium that causes Legionnaires' Disease.

The patient should be nursed in a position he finds comfortable. The physiotherapist should be requested to give the patient chest physiotherapy and to teach him breathing exercises. A cough linctus may be helpful. Sputum should be expectorated into a pot with a lid or disposable paper handkerchiefs. If the patient has active pulmonary tuberculosis, he should wear a high-efficiency filtration rate mask if he has to leave his room.

Respiratory therapy equipment, whether it be a simple inhaler, an oxygen humidifier or a respirator machine, will become contaminated both by the organisms in the patient's respiratory tract and by other opportunists such as Gram-negative bacteria which readily colonise warm, moist reservoirs. A procedure to eliminate these hazards must be implemented (see page 103).

Oral Hygiene

The patient with AIDS is particularly vulnerable to 'thrush' infection, caused by the yeast-like fungus *Candida albicans*. This infection commonly begins in the mouth but may quickly spread down the oesophagus or into the lungs. Frequent and careful oral hygiene is essential to keep the mouth clean and prevent such infections. The nurse should reinforce the importance of brushing the teeth after any food has been eaten. Disinfectant mouthwashes may be given to supplement this. If the patient is unconscious, his mouth should be cleaned at least every 2 hours and more often if necessary.

The nurse should inspect the patient's mouth twice a day. A torch and tongue depressor are essential. Kaposi's sarcoma lesions may first present in the mouth. Any sign of infection, such as white plaques, blisters or ulcers, should be reported to the doctor. Appropriate specimens will be obtained for investigations.

Toothache and dental caries should be remedied promptly.

Skin Care

Folliculitis is a common problem in a patient with AIDS. Various preparations for topical application may be prescribed.

It is not unusual for the patient to suffer from profuse night sweats. The skin should be kept clean and dry. Excessive drying can be countered by adding emollients to the water or by the application of body lotion. Linen and clothes should be changed as often as necessary.

The patient's peri-anal area may be sore as a result of excessive diarrhoea or because of intercurrent infection such as genital herpes or anal warts.

The patient's risk of developing pressure sores should be assessed using the Norton Score. Preventive measures that have been scientifically proven should be employed.

The nurse should observe the skin for signs of rashes. These may be due to drug reactions, or to infections such as herpes zoster (shingles) or chicken-pox. Kaposi's sarcoma manifests with skin lesions which vary considerably in appearance from small flat bruises to raised mauve plaques.

Wound Care

A wound is a breach in the first line of defence against infection: the intact skin. Micro-organisms can therefore gain access to sterile tissues and may initiate infection. Wounds caused by central or peripheral venous cannulation allow direct access of micro-organisms to the blood stream. These and other surgical incisions such as lymph node or skin biopsy sites must be treated with aseptic technique.

Pyrexia of Unknown Origin

A raised temperature may be the first sign of infection. This should be reported promptly to the doctor so that investigations can be initiated to determine the cause. Any invasive device such as an indwelling bladder catheter or intravenous infusion line should always be considered as a possible focus of infection. If implicated, it should be removed, because antibiotic therapy is unlikely to succeed in the presence of an infected device.

The patient's condition will determine how often and where the temperature should be recorded. Antipyretics such as aspirin may be given to help lower a temperature which is raised owing to pyrogens. Fanning the patient will not accomplish this, and such a measure may make the patient feel very uncomfortable.

Psychological Care

The psychological care of the patient is covered in detail elsewhere (see Chapter 7). The nurse should be aware that the disease process of AIDS may cause the patient's behaviour to alter. Infection of the central nervous system such as meningitis caused by the fungus *Cryptococcus neoformans* may give the patient a severe headache and photophobia. These symptoms may make him intolerant and aggressive. A sensitive, quiet approach is essential.

Terminal Care

The patient should be assured of a pain-free and dignified death. After death, certain precautions must be instituted during the care and removal of the infected body (see page 104).

HEALTH AND SAFETY OF STAFF

General Health

Staff who are themselves suffering from an infection such as herpes and those with weeping eczema or similar skin conditions should not care for these patients. Cuts and abrasions on hands and forearms must be covered with waterproof dressings. Staff exposed to AIDS patients and other patients with HTLV-III antibodies should be given the opportunity to volunteer blood samples for long-term storage (see page 59).

Protective Clothing

Disposable plastics aprons and latex gloves should be worn when exposed to blood or saliva — e.g. in venepuncture, mouth care, tracheal suction, cleaning up spillages of body fluids. A high-efficiency filtration rate face mask (theatre type) should be worn if the patient has active pulmonary tuberculosis.

During surgery, scrubbed staff should wear sterile disposable waterproof gowns (e.g. Convertors) in addition to other normal theatre attire. Eye protection BS 2092 should be worn by those who do not wear glasses if splashing into the conjunctivae is possible. Staff who transport the patient to and from theatre or other departments do not need to wear extra protective clothing, unless instructed by the nurse in charge of the ward or department.

Sharps Disposal

The prevention of 'needle-stick' injuries by the safe handling and disposal of 'sharps' is the *single most important way to prevent blood-to-blood spread* of the HTLV-III virus in the health care setting. A screw-capped evacuated blood collection system can be used for venepuncture – e.g. Exotainer. Needles must *not* be resheathed after use, as most inoculation accidents are caused by this procedure.

When conventional syringes and needles are used, the needle must not be snapped off the syringe, as this practice creates an aerosol hazard. The syringe and needle should be discarded into a sharps container which conforms to DHSS standard – e.g. CinBin. This is available in several sizes to meet the needs of community and hospital staff ($4\frac{1}{2}$ in size for district nurses, 1 gallon size for health centres, 2 gallon size for wards).

Scalpel blades must not be removed with the fingers. A device called Protectors can be used which removes the scalpel blade off the handle and also serves as a receiver for suture needles used during surgery.

Sharps containers must be burnt in an incinerator in the hospital or nearest health centre.

Specimens

All specimens should be handled in accordance with the ACDP Guidelines. Laboratory and portering staff must be alerted to the infectious nature of the specimens. Specimen containers and request cards must be labelled with 'Bio-Hazard' stickers. Lids must be securely fastened to prevent leakage in transit. The container and card are placed in separate compartments of a plastics envelope specimen bag, which, in turn, is placed in a leak-proof, autoclavable transport box.

Spillages

Spillages of blood or blood-stained secretions should be dealt with immediately. Sodium hypochlorite 1% (10 000 parts per million) is poured onto paper towels, which are placed over the spill. More solution is then gently poured on top. In the community, bleach 10% diluted 1 part bleach to 10 parts warm water can be used. If practical, the disinfectant is left for 30 min before being wiped up by the nurse, who wears disposable gloves and apron. (N.B.: Bleach rots fabrics and corrodes metals, so it should be used with care.) Towels, gloves and apron are then discarded as recommended for infected waste (see page 101).

Breakages

Clearing up glass presents a particular hazard, especially if specimen containers are broken. Household gloves (e.g. Marigold) must be worn. The pieces are wrapped up well in paper and discarded as recommended for infected waste. Hypochlorite is used if blood spillage occurred.

Inoculation Accident

In the event of an inoculation accident, the affected site should be 'milked', to encourage bleeding. The wound should be washed immediately with soap and water. Splashes of blood on the skin should also be washed off immediately with soap and water. Splashes of blood into the eyes or mouth should be irrigated with copious amounts of water or saline at the nearest eye-wash station. Eye-wash bottles (Contactasol) are available from the Occupational Health Department.

The staff member should seek medical advice at the earliest opportunity, either from the Occupational Health Department or from his or her own general practitioner. An accident form should be completed and the immediate superior notified.

Visits to Other Departments

If the patient has to visit another department for an investigation, the departmental staff must be advised, by telephone, of any precautions which may be necessary if they are likely to be exposed to blood or other infectious matter — e.g. faeces of *Salmonella* carriers. Such advance warning gives the staff time to activate their specific departmental policy. Supplies such as disinfectants and special equipment may need to be obtained. In addition, a 'Bio-Hazard' label should be stuck on the request card.

Maintenance Work in Wards/Departments

It is essential that staff from the Works Department are not exposed to unnecessary infection hazard. Before signing a 'permit to work', the nurse in charge must be satisfied that the area has been adequately decontaminated. If necessary, advice should be sought before allowing maintenance work to be carried out.

Laundry

Linen that is stained with blood or semen, or otherwise fouled or infected, should be heat disinfected by laundering at 95°C for 10 min. In hospital, linen is placed in a soluble plastics bag, inside a red plastics bag. The soluble bag is placed, unopened, into the designated washing machine. Because the linen is not sorted, this system prevents the laundry staff being put at risk. In the community, clothes can be washed in a domestic washing machine or the district nurse can arrange a special service.

Cleaning

The principles of cleaning are the same in the home as in the hospital. Hot water and detergent is used to remove dirt and grease from floors, fixtures and fittings. Cream cleanser is used to clean the sink, basins, toilet, shower or bath. In hospital, disposable cloths are used and discarded daily. Mop-heads are detachable and laundered daily. Mop buckets and bowls are emptied, washed and dried after use. Surfaces that have been contaminated with blood can be wiped over with sodium hypochlorite 0.1% (household bleach 10% diluted, 1 part bleach to 100 parts warm water). Crockery and cutlery can be washed in a dishwasher if available (hot wash cycle) or hand washed in hot (hand-hot) soapy water.

CLINICAL WASTE DISPOSAL

The national colour coding system for the disposal of clinical waste should be followed (Health Services Advisory Committee, 1982).

Infected Waste

Waste contaminated with blood or saliva must be discarded into yellow plastics bags and burnt. Special collections can be arranged by the district nurse for patients being nursed at home.

Non-infected Waste

Non-infected waste is discarded into black plastics bags and collected by the local borough council cleansing department.

Urine and Faeces

After use, the toilet is flushed in the usual way. Disinfectants are not necessary. If the patient used a bedpan or urinal, the equipment is either (a) disinfected with heat at 80°C for 1 min in the bedpan washing machine before being returned to communal use or (b) discarded into the macerator machine. The lid should be kept closed for 1 min after the cycle has stopped, to allow aerosols to settle.

MEDICAL/SURGICAL EQUIPMENT

Disposables should be used whenever possible. Re-usable equipment which has been contaminated with blood or saliva must be sterilised after use.

Sterilisation by heat is preferred, but chemicals or gas will have to be used for heat-labile equipment. Autoclaving is a commonly used method for heat sterilization:

$134°C$ for 3 min at 2.1 kg/cm^2 (220.8 kPa)
or
$121°C$ for 15 min at 1.05 kg/cm^2 (103 kPa)

Chemical sterilisation can be achieved with freshly activated buffered glutaraldehyde 2% for 3 h. (N.B.: This chemical is an irritant. Gloves, mask and eye protection must be worn when handling it. The room in which it is being used must be well ventilated.)

Ethylene oxide can be used for gas sterilisation:

Temperature $20–56°C$; humidity 50–60%; time 10 h; aeration 24 h

Central Sterile Supply Department (CSSD)/Theatre Sterile Supply Unit (TSSU)

The following precautions must be observed when returning equipment to CSSD or TSSU for reprocessing:

(1) Sharp instruments and breakables, such as scissors, forceps and glass bottles, must be placed in a stout container (e.g. Cobox).
(2) All equipment must be labelled 'Bio-Hazard'.
(3) The equipment must be mechanically washed in a washing machine before it is checked and sorted by hand.
(4) The equipment is then autoclaved.

Operating Departments

Some operating departments are not supplied by a TSSU and are responsible for processing their own equipment. In departments where there is no automated washing process, instruments and equipment must be autoclaved before being washed by hand. A solution such as Haemasol will be needed to remove blood. After thorough cleaning, the equipment is then sterilised by further autoclaving.

Fibre Optics

Fibre optics will be damaged by heat sterilisation. They should be chemically sterilised with glutaraldehyde. Automatic washing machines and purpose-built trolleys are commercially available. To reduce the risk of infection to staff who have to care for this equipment by hand, the following procedure is recommended.

Stage 1: Decontamination

Immerse for 1 h in freshly activated, buffered glutaraldehyde 2%. Discard solution.

Stage 2: Clean

Wash thoroughly with detergent and warm water. Air channels must be well irrigated. Rinse thoroughly.

Stage 3: Sterilise

Immerse for 3 h in a fresh solution of freshly activated, buffered glutaraldehyde 2%. Rinse thoroughly.

Mattress and Pillows

Protect with nylon proofed (impermeable) covers. Wash with warm soapy water when soiled and on discharge of patient.

Proctoscopes

Single-use disposables should be used and then incinerated.

Respiratory Therapy Equipment

Anaesthetic face mask and tubing: autoclave after use.
    Humidifier/nebuliser: single-use disposables, or, if re-usables are used, autoclave daily. Refill with sterile distilled water.
    Oxygen mask and tubing: change daily (sooner if soiled) and on discharge of patient.
    Simple inhaler and mouthpiece: autoclave after each treatment.
    Ventilators: protect with disposable siliconised filters. Use totally detachable circuits. Autoclave daily.

Suction Equipment

Suction canisters lined with plastics disposable containers (e.g. Receptal) are preferred. After use, the containers are sealed, placed in a bucket and carried by a porter to the incinerator. Non-disposable suction bottles and lids should be autoclaved at least daily and on discharge of the patient. The contents are emptied out down the sluice carefully, to avoid splashes. When in use, 100 ml sodium hypochlorite 1% is poured into the bottle. Suction tubing must be changed daily and on discharge of the patient.

Thermometers

Protect with a plastics disposable sleeve (e.g. Dispotemp). After use, invaginate, and discard into yellow plastics bag for incineration.

SOCIAL SERVICES

Social Workers

Social workers do not need to wear any protective clothing to shake hands and talk to the patient.

Meals on Wheels

Those who deliver the meals do not need to wear any protective clothing when they go into the patient's home. It is quite safe to handle money that is given in return for the food.

Home Care Team/Home Helps and Other Supporting Agencies

For health and safety, and protective clothing, see page 98.

Social Clubs and Pubs

Patients should not be excluded from eating and drinking on these premises.

Religious Services

Patients should not be excluded from participating in services at their chosen place of worship. There is no evidence of infection being transmitted by a communal communion chalice.

Public Library

Books that have been borrowed do not require any special treatment.

Domestic Premises

Furniture that has been used by the patient does not require any special treatment — i.e. sofas, mattresses and pillows do not need to be burnt. The house does not require 'fumigation'.

CARE AND REMOVAL OF THE INFECTED BODY

Advice on the precautions necessary for the safe handling of the body should be sought from any member of the Infection Control Team. There are specific rules which must be followed for handling the cadaver in the isolation room, mortuary and coffin.

PROCEDURE AFTER DEATH

(1) The body must not be handled unnecessarily.

(2) Staff who perform last offices should wear the appropriate protective clothing, viz. disposable plastics apron, unsterile disposable latex gloves.

(3) If, for religious reasons, an attendant is required to handle the body, the nurse in charge should explain the infectious hazard before issuing the appropriate protective clothing. However, this should be strongly discouraged.

(4) The infected body must be enclosed in a plastics cadaver bag before it is transported to the mortuary. If the patient dies at home, the GP advises the undertaker to provide this.

(5) Relatives and close friends should be encouraged to view the body *before* removal from the ward/house. This facility will not be possible at the undertakers, and it is *extremely* difficult to arrange viewing once the body has been taken to the hospital mortuary. Arrangements must be made with the consultant histopathologist.

(6) *Escorted* viewing, in the Chapel of Rest, can only be organised under extenuating circumstances.

(7) Members of the chaplaincy are always available to offer support to the bereaved. This includes escorting to view the body.

(8) On no account must the cadaver bag be unzipped.

(9) *Last Offices*

    (a) Straighten the body; close the eyes and mouth.

    (b) Unless it is a coroner's case, remove drips, drains, tubes, catheters, etc. Discard immediately into yellow plastic bags and knot them.

    (c) Discard sharps into sharps bin.

    (d) Seal all leaking wounds with occlusive dressings.

    (e) Pack leaking orifices.

    (f) Only wash those parts of the body that are grossly soiled.

    (g) Attach identity bracelets to ankle and wrist. (N.B.: They should be secured in such a way that they can be read through the transparent plastics bag for identification purposes.)

    (h) Label the body with 'Bio-Hazard – Danger of Infection' tape.[1] This can be placed around the ankle and around the wrist.

    (i) Put paper shroud on the body, then place body in plastics cadaver bag.[2]

    (j) Attach 'Notification of Death' label to outside of plastics cadaver bag with 'Bio-Hazard – Danger of Infection' tape. This alerts the mortuary staff to the danger of infection.

    (k) Discard all infected linen into soluble bags within red plastics bags. Knot them.

    (l) Discard all protective clothing and rubbish into yellow plastics bags and knot them.

(m) A porter who has been specifically trained in the safety precuations necessary will handle linen and dispose of waste.

(10) Porters transporting the body to the mortuary (or the mortuary ambulance crew) are not required to wear protective clothing, because the cadaver bag acts as a barrier to the dissemination of the infectious agent. An infected body must be placed, feet first, in one of the designated fridges. Only infected bodies should be placed in these compartments.

(11) A large notice saying 'Danger of Infection' is fixed on the appropriate doors of the body store.

(12) The advice of the consultant histopathologist must be sought before a post-mortem examination is carried out. As a general rule, post mortems are not performed on cases or suspected cases of AIDS except under the conditions approved by the Dangerous Pathogens Advisory Group. If a post mortem is carried out, then attendants need to wear appropriate protective clothing and follow the procedure specified in the appropriate Code of Practice (Department of Health and Social Security, 1978).

(13) Undertakers will be advised to supply a 'finished leak-proof coffin' and be required to sign a 'Notice of Infection' supplied by the mortuary staff.

(14) The body should not be embalmed or otherwise injected by the undertakers.

Equipment Notes

1. The 'Bio-Hazard — Danger of Infection' tape is available in rolls 66 m long from Jencons (Scientific) Ltd, Leighton Buzzard, Bucks., UK.
2. The clear plastics cadaver bags with zip around three sides are manufactured by Syrein Plastics Ltd: £5.00 + VAT.

APPENDIX

Useful Information for Patients

(1) The long-term prognosis for an individual infected with HTLV-III is unknown. However, data available from studies conducted among homosexual men who are HTLV-III-antibody-positive indicate that most persons will remain infected, but only 5-20% will develop AIDS within 2-5 years (Curran, 1985).

(2) Although asymptomatic, these individuals may transmit HTLV-III to others. Regular medical evaluation and follow-up is advised, especially for individuals who develop signs or symptoms suggestive of AIDS or other related disorders.

(3) There is a risk of infecting others by sexual intercourse. The efficacy of condoms in preventing infection with HTLV-III is unproven, but the consistent use of them may reduce transmission. Tests are being undertaken on extra-strong sheaths.

(4) Although there is a possibility of infection via saliva through oral–genital contact or intimate kissing, the risk from saliva during ordinary social contact is negligible.

(5) Women with a sero-positive test or women whose sexual partner is sero-positive are themselves at increased risk of developing AIDS. If they become pregnant, their offspring are also at increased risk of developing AIDS.

(6) Those who are HTLV-III-antibody-positive must refrain from donating blood, plasma, body organs, other tissue and sperm.

(7) There is a risk to other intravenous drug abusers through the sharing of needles, syringes and mixing bowls. Disposable needles and syringes should always be used if possible. They must be used once only and then discarded into a stout container and burnt. If glass syringes have to be used (by, for example, diabetics), the parts should be separated and placed in a container with a tightly fitting lid (e.g. saucepan), completely covered with water and boiled for 5 min.

(8) Toothbrushes, razors or other implements that could become contaminated with blood should not be shared.

(9) Tampons can be flushed down the toilet.

(10) Sanitary towels must be burnt. If this cannot be achieved in the house (coal fire, bonfire), the district nurse will arrange appropriate collection for incineration along with other infected waste.

(11) Clothes and linen that are stained with blood or semen should be washed in a washing machine at 95°C for 10 min or boiled before hand washing.

(12) Crockery and cutlery can be hand washed with hot soapy water (hand-hot) or in a dishwasher.

(13) When seeking any medical or dental care, patients/clients should inform those responsible for their care of their positive antibody status so that appropriate evaluation can be undertaken and precautions taken to prevent transmission to others. The hospital may be able to provide a list of dental practitioners who have agreed to treat those who are HTLV-III-antibody-positive.

(14) The Terrence Higgins Trust is a registered charity which provides an advisory service for those suffering from AIDS and related disorders.

Address: BM AIDS,
London WC1N 3XX
Tel. no.: 01 278 8745

Registered Trade Marks

Convertors:	American Hospital Supply Corporation
Exotainer:	Labco Ltd
CinBin:	Labco Ltd
Protectors:	Richards
Marigold:	LRC Products Ltd
Contactasol:	Contactasol Ltd
Cobox:	Sterilin Medical Ltd

Haemosol: Meinecke & Co. Inc., Baltimore
Receptal: Sorenson Research Co. Inc.
Dispotemp: Anstro-Sjuco U.K.

REFERENCES

Advisory Committee on Dangerous Pathogens (1984). *Acquired Immune Defic-iency Syndrome (AIDS) – Interim Guidelines*
Communicable Disease Report 84/52. PHLS Communicable Disease Surveillance Centre
Curran, James W. (1985). Opening Address, *International Conference on Acquired Immune Deficiency Syndrome*, Atlanta, Georgia, 15 April 1985
Department of Health and Social Security (1978). *Code of Practice for the Prevention of Infection in Clinical Laboratories and Post-Mortem Rooms.* London, HMSO
Health Services Advisory Committee (1982). *The Safe Disposal of Clinical Waste.* HMSO, London

PART 2: NURSING MANAGEMENT OF IN-PATIENTS

INTRODUCTION

For nursing purposes, the various diagnostic groups (AIDS, ARC, PGL, sero-positive)* are divided into two practical management groups of patients:

(1) Those who are seriously ill and require admission for intensive treatment of a complication either within the AIDS diagnosis or arising from the AIDS-related complex (ARC). In general, this group is best cared for in single rooms within a complex that specialises in their care. This approach has the advantage of controlling and rationalising all skills and equipment as well as meeting the specific requirements mentioned on page 94. Most of the following recommendations for nursing management of in-patients relate to this group.

(2) (a) Those who are sero-positive and are acutely ill because of some other (non-HTLV-III-related) cause, or (b) those who are sero-positive with or without PGL who are not acutely ill and require hospital investigations. This second group is usually nursed in the ward or other clinical area that specialises in the specific treatment or investigation required. It is necessary, therefore, that all nurses within a receiving hospital have a working knowledge of nursing and control of infection procedures for these patients.

A few points should be made regarding the nursing management of sero-positive and PGL patients in the general wards.

*Diagnostic groups are defined and classified in Chapter 1.

General Ward Care

A single room should be made available but is not essential for PGL and sero-positive patients. It is an advantage to protect these patients from being in the public eye. All nursing care should be carried out according to the hospital's Hepatitis B Control of Infection Procedure. Ward staff (including domestic staff) should be quite clear as to how the patient is to be managed. There must be no lack of clarity but also no breaking of confidence. It is extremely important to the PGL and sero-positive patients that they are not confused with patients who have received the diagnosis of AIDS. They are often very anxious and very knowledgeable about their diagnosis. They are living in hope that they do not develop AIDS.

Implications of HTLV-III-positive diagnosis are the same as those of a diagnosis of frank AIDS, with respect to sexual activity and personal control, and follow-up counselling by nursing staff should be predicated on an understanding of such implications for the patient (see Chapter 8).

TOTAL PATIENT CARE

The seriously ill AIDS and ARC patients require a full range of nursing care. Table 6.1 is a guide to the major problem areas that both patient and nurse are likely to meet.

To illustrate the problems commonly encountered, four medical histories are presented, with nursing comment.

Case 1

A 34-year-old homosexual with a history of syphilis and gonorrhoea was a known contact of an AIDS patient, with a stable monogamous relationship. He attended the STD clinic from the time he was known to be an AIDS contact. Initially he was well, but developed diarrhoea, loss of weight and general malaise. *Shigella flexneri* was found in his stool. Concurrently he developed a herpes infection of the peri-anal and scrotal areas. He was treated as an out-patient with oral acyclovir, amphotericin lozenges, ketoconazole and codeine phosphate.

Four days after commencing the codeine phosphate, he developed an ataxia for which he was admitted as an in-patient. On withdrawal of codein phosphate the ataxia rapidly resolved. His CT scan was normal. He was discharged home on antifungal treatment.

He was admitted 6 months later with a fever, dry cough and worsening watery diarrhoea. At sigmoidoscopy a biopsy showed CMV colitis; foscarnet was prescribed. Septrin was prescribed for an assumed *Pneumocystis carinii* pneumonia, but bronchial washings (taken prior to septrin therapy) did not show *Pneumocystis carinii* or acid-fast bacilli but *Mycobacterium xenopi* was found on culture. He began to show neurological signs of brain-stem damage. He

Table 6.1

Problem	Desired outcomes	Nursing action
Anxiety due to: lack of knowledge of illness effect of illness on activities of daily living (ADL), including sexual activities dying	Verbalise anxiety Sleep at night	(1) Give information required – inform team (2) Use correct agency – doctor, psychologist, health adviser, dietician and social worker (3) Practical help – home care (dependents and pets); will; money worries; housing (4) Relationships – arrange contact of friends and/or relatives (that patient needs to see) (5) Minor tranquillisers/night sedation – assess need regular/p.r.n.
Anger due to: anticipated loss of life less quality of life due to injustice (e.g. perceived lack of care)	Less displacement of anger Verbalise anger	(1) Give time, sit and listen; allow venting of anger (2) Where justified or where quality of life can be improved, adjust care and inform team (3) Use psychologist
Depression due to: reaction to specific problems reaction to impending loss of everybody and everything	Verbalise fears and guilt Become socially responsive	(1) Give information as needed (2) Help solve specific problem – e.g. job, wife (3) Relieve underlying guilt – sit and listen (4) Silent/passive presence (5) Observation/not forced interaction (6) Referral to psychologist

Susceptibility to infection due to: immune deficiency (absolute reduction in numbers of T helper lymphocytes) repeated opportunist infection antibiotic therapy malnutrition

No signs or symptoms of infection
Behavioural evidence of patient's ability to prevent infection
Minimal dependence on antibiotic, antifungal and antiviral agents

(1) Provide protective isolation – single room with washing and toilet facilities en suite

(2) Appropriate hand washing for attendants, visitors and patient(s)

(3) Constant explanation to increase understanding of methods of avoiding infection

(4) Ensure complete diet – consult dietician

(5) Monitor vital signs 4-hourly

(6) Daily assessment of lungs, mouth, GU tract, rectum/anus and skin; culture as appropriate; monitor temperature 1–4-hourly

(7) If temperature rises, notify doctor, give antipyretics as prescribed (assess prescription); use fan carefully

(8) Mouth care 1–4-hourly – soft atraumatic toothbrush and toothpaste ± soda bicarbonate and salt

(9) Peri-anal care – wash and dry carefully after stool

(10) Use external urinary drainage systems where possible; when indwelling catheters are used, ensure closed drainage and aseptic procedure

Table 6.1 (cont'd)

Problem	Desired outcomes	Nursing action
Nausea, vomiting, diarrhoea and constipation due to: intestinal parasite – e.g. cytomegalovirus (CMV) GI involvement of Kaposi's sarcoma chemotherapy antibiotic regimen radiotherapy electrolyte imbalance	Normal skin turgor No nausea, vomiting or diarrhoea Stop loss of weight Obtain increase in weight Normal fluid balance Mucous membranes soft No signs or symptoms of electrolyte imbalance	(1) Enteric precautions; private room, toilet and shower when possible; gloves and apron when handling secretions (2) Nil by mouth, diet as tolerated and per order of dietician (3) Fluid balance chart, daily weights, abdominal girth once a day if indicated (4) Assess bowel sounds q.d.s. (5) Quantitative stool and nasogastric (NG) output; note quality (colour, consistency) (6) Assess hydration, skin turgor, mucous membranes (7) Mouth care 1–4 hourly; ice cubes as tolerated (8) Administer antiemetics, antidiarrhoeals and stool-softening agents; assess need for changes to prescription (9) Maintain NG patency and position, irrigate p.r.n. (10) Dietary consultation, calorie count, if appropriate (11) Special handling of blood samples for serum electrolytes (12) Total parenteral nutrition (see Appendix) – aseptic care of i.v. cannula and lines

Respiratory distress due to:
chest infection caused by *Pneumocystis carinii, Candida*
pleural effusions
Kaposi's lesions of bronchial tree

Breath sounds clear, denies shortness of breath (SOB)
No cough
Able to carry out ADLs without distress

(1) Assess
(2) Monitor temperature, pulse, respiration and overall physical assessment (especially energy expended in breathing)
(3) Position patient for greatest comfort (least energy expended)
(4) Teach proper coughing and deep breathing technique; encourage 2–4-hourly
(5) Incentive spirometer when indicated
(6) Encourage use of O_2 and humidification when ordered
(7) Procure specimens when cough is productive – utilise postural drainage
(8) Special handling of arterial blood samples for gases and recording of results

Weakness and fatigue due to:
inadequate nutrition
anaemia
malabsorption
increased metabolic demands (fevers and disease)
radiotherapy
exhausting tests and investigations

Able to perform ADLs without SOB or fatigue
Pulse 100/min or less

(1) Plan activities within limits of patient's tolerance; assist p.r.n.
(2) Refer to physiotherapist as appropriate
(3) Arrange environment for optimum convenience – e.g. accessibility of bedside, commode and hand basin
(4) Assess and treat loose stools, constipation, incontinence and vomiting
(5) Assess for shortness of breath and general mobility
(6) Encourage lover and/or family to assist patient

Table 6.1 (cont'd)

Problem	Desired outcomes	Nursing action
		(7) Reassure patient of continual assistance and support; give information
		(8) Massage and comforting non-verbal communication
		(9) Plan for continuing care/convalescence
Skin breakdown due to: diarrhoea oedema immobility dietary insufficiency	Skin intact No breakdown Verbalised comfort Maximum possible mobility	(1) Avoid pressure on extremities
		(2) Careful examination of potential breakdown areas, particularly sacral area and scrotum
		(3) Assess oedema for increase; measure girths when indicated
		(4) Consider fibre mattress, water and low-air-loss beds, sheepskin, cradle, etc.
		(5) Decubitus care; enlist surgical clinical nurse specialist as indicated
		(6) Shower and thorough washing
		(7) Position change 1–4 h with pillows
		(8) Ambulate when able; up in chair
		(9) Check completeness of diet
Pain due to: abdominal cramping	Able to verbalise pain and need for painkillers; pain controlled by analgesia	(1) Analgesia as ordered; evaluate effectiveness

oedema, ascites
persistent coughing
decubitus breakdown
mucusitis
long-term NG placement
multiple procedures
fear of the unknown
fear of loss of identity
loneliness
catastrophe – e.g. perforated bowel

or alternative treatment
Relaxed expression and position
Restful sleep

(2) Consider need for schedule as opposed to p.r.n. and frequency, dosage and drug type changes
(3) Medicate prior to ambulatory procedures
(4) Assist with position changes; position for comfort
(5) Scrotal support; TEDs
(6) Consider need for i.v. pump analgesia; titrate for adequate control
(7) Supplement with sedatives, antianxiety medicines and techniques as required
(8) Teach and assist patient and family with alternative methods of relaxation – i.e. visualisation and massage
(9) Diversionary activity; out of room when possible; TV and radio
(10) Reassure patient; when possible be with patient and recognise physical and mental, emotional and spiritual pain

Confusion, ataxia, dysphasia, dysphagia, paralysis, parathaesia (and depression) due to:
AIDS encephalopathy
cerebral involvement of toxoplasmosis, herpes, CMV, etc.

Regain specific function
Prevent deterioration/complications
Obtain maximum mobility

(1) Administer antibiotics, antivirals and antifungal agents
(2) Assess regularly level of consciousness and gross motor and sensory abilities
(3) Protect patient p.r.n. – e.g. low bed; darkened room; cot sides; padding on floor; frequent check visits

Table 6.1 *(cont'd)*

Problem	Desired outcomes	Nursing action
		(4) Consult physiotherapist; programme for maximum mobility; teach nurses, patient and relatives
		(5) Increase frequency of turning, passive exercises and basic hygiene p.r.n.
		(6) Give medication for anxiety, depression and pain (see under 'Anxiety', 'Depression' and 'Pain')

Nursing criteria for discharge of maintenance (overall expected outcomes)

(1) Patient can state what the plans are for future care – i.e. return to clinic, tests, chemotherapy, etc.

(2) Patient demonstrates ability and has resources to care for self at home.

(3) Lover and/or family are prepared for homecoming.

(4) Community nursing/hospice nurse has made assessment and is available as appropriate.

(5) Other agencies are informed of intended discharge – e.g. out-patient's department, GP and referring physician.

(6) Continuing treatment and investigations are planned and appointments made.

became very dyspnoeic, exhausted and confused, with increasing basal shadowing and effusions on X-ray. He was transferred to the Intensive Care Unit, where he was mechanically ventilated, and died 3 days later, just 19 days after admission.

Comment

Initially his breathing was best aided by laying him nearly flat and on his side. Physiotherapy was commenced early but no sputum was obtained. Oxygen was delivered via an Accuroex mask, first at 28% and then later at 40% and 60% to meet an ever-decreasing partial pressure of oxygen in arterial blood (samples taken). In the Intensive Care Unit he required postural drainage and percussion as well as vibration. He was mechanically ventilated and required very frequent endotracheal suction for copious secretions.

The constant challenge of watery diarrhoea to peri-anal tissues and sacral pressure areas was successfully countered with application of E45 cream. Although in considerable discomfort, he remained calm until he became confused. He appeared to develop an acceptance, not of death but of the disease. His lover visited him daily and stayed almost continuously during the last 10 days. The patient had told his mother about his homosexuality and his disease. His mother also stayed throughout most of his last admission. His mother and lover supported each other as well as him. The medical decision to take the patient to the Intensive Care Unit was based on the fact that specific antibiotic therapy was started late in the course of the pneumonia; it was thought imperative to maintain him for a few days to allow the antibiotic therapy to have effect. Both the patient's mother and lover were hopeful initially, but began to suffer grief and loss when he commenced mechanical ventilation. They found considerable consolation in each other's company when he died.

Case 2

A 45-year-old male homosexual who had multiple sexual contacts over 20 years, all of whom had been British except one from North America. He had been treated for serum hepatitis (B surface-antigen-positive) syphilis and gonorrhoea in the past. In the 4 years prior to his admission he had recurrent episodes of peri-anal herpes simplex. He began to lose weight (30 kg in approximately 8 months) before a diagnosis of AIDS was made. He developed lethargy and malaise but no lymphadenopathy.

He was admitted for treatment of a *Pneumocystis carinii* chest infection which was diagnosed from bronchoscopy (bronchial lavage and washings). He was treated with high-dosage oral septrin followed by trimethoprin alone. He also suffered from oro-oesophageal candidiasis (Ba swallow was used to confirm diagnosis), which was treated with nystatin topically and ketoconazole systemically. His appetite improved and he stopped losing weight (now 54 kg). It was noted that on occasion he was a little vague. There were no abnormalities found on CT scan, EEG and lumbar puncture.

He was admitted 6 weeks later with what was described as giddiness and a sore eye. He was found to be ataxic and to have a fungal infection of the retina. He commenced treatment with 5-flucytosine and amphotericin intravenously. He developed severe rigors and pyrexia only while receiving amphotericin. His intellectual abilities began to deteriorate despite treatment. He became disorientated in time and space. His condition changed from hour to hour. His sight began to fail, first in one eye and then in the other. He developed a right hemiparesis which worsened. Another CT scan now showed multiple abscesses. After 10 days of antifungal treatment his toxoplasma dye test became positive. He began treatment with pyrimethamine and sulfadoxine for toxoplasmosis.

His neurological signs improved initially but then continually changed over a period of 3 weeks, with no further overall improvement.

After 1 month of treatment he became confused and incontinent, and began suffering severe pain in all limbs and his abdomen. A diamorphine infusion was commenced. He began fitting 10 days before he died. He was given phenobarbitone, which partially controlled the fits. He died almost exactly a year after onset of his first symptoms.

Comment

During his first admission he received care for a *Pneumocystis* chest infection as already described for Case 1.

His later admission was characterised by a high level of dependency on basic nursing care. His confusion, ataxia, hemiparesis and loss of sight made him more liable to falling. His bed was kept in a low position at all times that he was unattended. The single room was an advantage in terms of privacy during a very undignified period of illness, but frequent room checks were required to ensure comfort and safety.

Urinary incontinence was managed with the use of a Texas catheter and drainage bag. In the last 2 weeks he required continuous one-to-one nursing care. He required patience for successful communication and constant help with feeding, personal hygiene and mobility.

Case 3

A 32-year-old homosexual businessman. He had a stable relationship recently in the UK but had been to North America 2 years previously, where he had had 50 sexual contacts in 2 weeks and he also had a tattoo. He had no symptoms until he developed proctitis and diarrhoea. He stopped having sexual intercourse because of the colitis. He attended the STD clinic at his district general hospital, where he was found to have a gonococcal rectal infection, which was treated successfully. His diarrhoea persisted (twelve bowel movements a day consisting mainly of mucus). He lost 10 kg in weight. He was referred to a consultant physician, who diagnosed ulcerative colitis, for which he received standard medication, including steroids; frequency of bowel movement was reduced, but consistency of stool was still very abnormal.

Ten weeks after his diarrhoea began, he noticed purple spots on both feet, which progressively coalesced to form patches on the feet, and further developed over 6 months on legs, arms, abdomen and buttocks.

A further 8 weeks later he began to pass blood in his stool (eight times a day). Thirteen months after his first symptoms, both feet became swollen and he was referred to a dermatologist, who took biopsies — Kaposi's sarcoma (KS) was confirmed a week later. He was then referred to the STD clinic. He was found, although otherwise well, to have a reduced T helper lymphocyte cell population. He was admitted for a lymph node biopsy and was discovered to have KS of the bowel, lymph node and trachea. He was started on a course of alpha-interferon, to continue for 1 year.

He was readmitted for reassessment, and the KS lesions on his feet had returned to being discrete instead of confluent. However, he was found to have candidiasis in the nails and he had severe constipation, with blood and mucus. His lymph nodes were less enlarged than they had been but his sigmoid colon was rigid with tumour. He had developed a severe anaemia and was transfused for this. He went home for a few days. From this point on, he saw the possibility of not recovering and was very depressed on occasions. He returned with a dry cough and his temperature ranged diurnally from 36°C to 40°C for a few days. He had lost a further 6 kg since his admission. In view of the poor function of his bowel, he was offered radiotherapy, which was begun immediately.

On his third and final admission (approximately 20 months after the onset of his first symptoms), his legs became swollen and his bowel became worse, despite both alpha-interferon and radiotherapy. At first he felt well enough to go on week-end leave but later was too weak.

Almost exactly 2 years after the onset of his first symptoms, he developed acute peritonitis due to bowel perforation and he died 3 days afterwards.

Comment on Major Nursing Problems

He had periods of very high temperatures during the early part of his first admission. These were treated with paracetamol but occasionally tepid sponging was required in addition. Fanning was used, but only with great care; it was uncomfortable and needed to be intermittent to be effective. Although regular observations of temperature were increased to hourly for short periods, at other times it was essential that nurses took the initiative to touch his skin and enquire as to whether he felt hot or cold (both sensations required a thermometer measurement).

His initial diarrhoea was controlled by codeine phosphate. His anus became very sore. His rectum became tender. His stool became small and hard. Oral lactulose was given to soften his stool.

Owing to depression and resulting lethargy and abdominal pain, he scored a surprisingly low Norton Score early on his first admission. His skin was closely examined each day for changes to KS lesions and for pressure sores or occurrence of general folliculitis or eczema. Stomahesive was applied to the area from the sacrum to the perineum in order to reduce the effects of both incontinence and shearing.

Although time was given to sitting with him and he was allowed time to vent his feelings, the nursing staff were never able to gain his trust. He lied on several occasions. Most significantly, he lied about where he was staying and pretended that the people he lived with were his parents, thus distancing his real parents not only from knowledge of what was happening now, but also, perhaps more importantly, from his past and his sexuality.

Despite presenting with a dry cough and high temperature and being broncho-scoped twice (bronchial washing being sent for microscopy and culture), no opportunist infection of his lungs was ever found. He did not develop shortness of breath until very near to death. All he required was a little simple linctus to aid sleep at night.

Drinking and eating tended to increase the amount of abdominal cramping pain he experienced. He tolerated a bland low-fibre, frequent, small-portion diet. Salads and fruit gave rise to severe abdominal pain. Temgesic and Buscapan were given as required. However, despite these measures, he still suffered a great deal and continued to have small hard stools accompanied by blood and mucus and had his bowels open frequently and painfully. He received a continuous pump infusion of pethidine for pain during the last 36 h of his life.

Case 4

A 44-year-old bisexual married man. He was admitted with chronic diarrhoea, complaining of rapid weight loss after a month abroad. His diarrhoea was explosive (once an hour). He had a sore mouth (*Candida*). He had severe pyrexia (wearing three sweaters in a room temperature of 24 °C). CMV of the gut was diagnosed on a sigmoid biopsy. His treatment was as follows:

Candidiasis of mouth treated with nystatin suspension topically and ketoconazole systemically.

CMV of the gut treated with foscarnet.

Diarrhoea treated with loperamide and codeine phosphate, and bland and generally low-bulk diet.

E45 cream was used to maintain integrity of anal and peri-anal areas.

The diarrhoea continued despite all treatment. The patient abandoned the diet. His wife brought him in his favourite food (fruit, salmon and cakes), and he suffered. Gradually the diarrhoea subsided and he stopped losing weight. He went home for 2 months. He was readmitted with further loss of weight and continuing diarrhoea, and was treated with intravenous fluids and plasma. A high-calorie diet was begun and he regained his previous discharge weight (50 kg). His diarrhoea continued but he felt better and wished to go home.

He died 3 weeks later at home.

Comment

It is notable that this man did not inform his wife that he was bisexual and that he did not wish her to know that he had AIDS. This raised both practical and ethical problems for the nurses, but his wife remained attentive, unquestioning and untold of his diagnosis until his death.

In association with this lack of honesty with his wife, it is important to note that the patient reached a high level of acceptance of death. He died feeling that he had maintained control and protected his wife from additional pain.

MAJOR ISSUES

At present there are a few areas of great concern in relation to the nursing needs of AIDS in-patients. These will now be considered in some detail.

Dying, Death and Depression

Much is said elsewhere (e.g. Chapters 7 and 8) on the practical and psychological implications of diagnosis for the patient, and the sorts of decisions he may be required to face as a consequence. The nurse's role is to try and facilitate the thinking that goes on before major decisions regarding the consequences of diagnosis are made. The nurse needs to sit and listen and act as a sounding-board for the patient's proposals. She must never normally direct the patient or force the issue, otherwise she is likely to enhance a sense of powerlessness and inadequacy.

Warning having been given of the dangers of directing the patient in his decision making, it must be said that avoidance of the issues at hand is also unhelpful. If the patient asks what he should do, then alternatives should be discussed. The nurse, drawing on experience, should present all the alternatives she knows in as open and balanced a manner as possible: again the decision must come from the patient.

Practicalities of death need to be dealt with at appropriate times. It is perfectly reasonable for a nurse to ask whether the patient's will is in order when he is talking about the people he is going to leave behind him when he dies.

When the patient is depressed, it is useful to differentiate between the reactive and endogenous elements of his depression. The reactive elements can be elicited in terms of cause and effect, and the nurse can aid the patient through compassion and sensitivity.

A young male homosexual who has had to stop having sexual intercourse may be depressed at his loss of sexual prowess. He may be anxious that his lover will seek others for physical comfort. Compliments from the nurse as to his general good looks or a particularly attractive physical feature may help. It may also be worth while broaching the subject carefully with his lover and, if appropriate, discussing techniques for safe sex and the need for trust between them. His lover may also be anxiously depressed because he fears (or knows) that he is infected with the virus. The nurse must be extremely sensitive to both the patient's and his lover's individual needs. In order to increase mutual trust, it is generally good practice to give information to them both at the same time, to enhance a sense of sharing. However, great care must be taken not to break confidentiality with the patient and not to impose on his partner a role which he does not wish, or is unable, to accept. Both patient and lover may derive strength from shared hope of recovery; the nurse must avoid destroying this hope even if, in her view, it is unrealistic. She may help modify the hope as part of a team approach — for example, focus attention on the recovery from the present opportunistic infection rather than on the long-term outlook.

The endogenous element of depression is considered to be both a direct consequence of viral activity (AIDS encephalopathy) and the anticipative condition of looking forward to death and the loss of everyone and everything. When an AIDS sufferer's physical condition allows (i.e. where death is not imminent but endogenous depression is acute and severe), then he should undoubtedly be cared for in a mental health facility but visited as if he were at home*, in order to provide continuity of care.

When death is imminent, the nurse needs to provide comfort and distraction. Favourite music and videos may be used at the patient's discretion. He needs to be given only simple choices and decisions, and not many of them. It is often more acceptable for the nurse to hold the patient's hand, stroke his hair or offer him a well-chosen prayer or poem rather than expect him to converse with her. However, the nurse must not impose on her patient. Everyday routines should be within the patient's control as far as his negative feelings and lethargy will allow, and the nurse should take care to avoid 'over-nursing' — i.e. doing things for the patient that the patient can do for himself. The patient is often silent and socially unresponsive. Care must continue to be given unconditionally. The patient is usually more dependent on the nurses for activities of daily living, so the total nursing requirement is increased.

Special attention should be given to the patient's environment, pressure area care, mouth care, mood changes, eating and bowel habits. Suicide prevention should be implemented unobtrusively.

The nurse must not feel that it is failure on her part if the endogenous element of depression shows little sign of lifting. It has been our experience that few AIDS sufferers reach a state of verbalised acceptance of death.

The degree of spiritual development required of a patient to reach a state of acceptance of death is very great. Much of the strength for this development will come from the patient and the facilitative approach of the caring team. The nurse needs to discern the spiritual needs of the patient early on and assess them regularly. Some male homosexuals may feel indifferent, estranged or even hostile to the established church. However, it is essential that the hospital chaplains be

*See section on 'Management of AIDS Sufferer in the Community' (page 127).

offered and remain on offer as resource for the patient. In hospitals the chaplains are frequently the most experienced, most available counsellors in matters of dying and death. The chaplain should be regarded as a key member of the caring team if the patient so wishes.

The Patient's Visitors

The nurses must make visitors feel welcome. Forbidding signs on ward doors should be abandoned in favour of positive instructions for a successful visit. Visiting times should be organised as part of the care plan for the individual patient, with the sole intention of providing what is beneficial for the patient and his relationships with others; they should be constantly reviewed in the light of the patient's wishes and changing condition.

The lovers, wives, families and friends of AIDS patients play an important part in their psychological care. The relationship between the nurse and these people plays an important part in the welfare of the patient. The nurse should rapidly become aware that homosexual relationships may be as deep and meaningful as heterosexual relationships. Despite the law, lovers may regard each other as next-of-kin, and exclusion of a partner will cause great distress. It is vital that the nursing staff be guided by the patient's wishes but his lover will require counselling in his own right. He will be anxious about his own health as well as his partner's (the patient). He will need information and counselling, especially for grief, loss and bereavement. He may also exhibit anger that could be displaced towards staff or friends of the patient. He may experience guilt, which can be enhanced by fear of his being the source of infection. He should be offered the chance to take part in the care of his loved one where this is appropriate.

The nursing staff need to be aware of possible complications, especially when the patient is bisexual or has several concurrent sexual partners. The nurse may be confronted with a wife who may or may not know of her husband's infidelity, alternative life-style or the presence of a male lover. The nurse needs to handle the situation with tact and sympathy but within the limits of confidentiality set by the patient.

Friends of the patient should be encouraged to visit when possible, in order to give a broad base for emotional support of the patient. The patient can use different friends as counsellors for problems and elicit a range of reactions; this can often facilitate decision making for the patient. However, the nurse must be guided by the patient when disclosing information to friends. It may be that the patient wishes only selected people to be given information; and in order to maintain a close, trusting relationship between patient and nurse, it is imperative that his wishes be carried out.

The parental family may be faced with the triple shock of discovering, within a short period of time, that son or brother is an active homosexual, that he has AIDS and that he is dying. In particular, parents may experience an additional sense of loss in the knowledge of their son's previous exclusion of them from an important part of his life. It has been our experience that the patient may continue to conduct his life in two separate compartments even while he is dying. The nurse needs to support parents and siblings as well as the patient. She must let them vent feelings of anger, which may be displaced and projected at their son's lover, and guilt that they have done something wrong and caused the 'abnormality of homosexuality' in their son or brother. Background information is often helpful, and organisations such as Gay Switchboard, charities or self-help groups are useful supplements to information from the caring team.

Clinical Nurse

Development

The skills demanded of the nurse supporting the AIDS patient are many and varied. Previous experience of high-dependency and psychiatric nursing as well as the nursing of dying and STD patients would all clearly be most useful. However, it is unlikely that all these skill areas can be combined in one person, but it is possible to combine them within the team. The main areas of skill and knowledge development that will be required by all nurses are as follows.

(1) The nurse's knowledge of AIDS must be thorough and extensive. It must be continually updated. Both *Morbidity and Mortality Weekly Report* and *Communicable Disease Report* (see References and Bibliography) are useful sources of recent developments.

(2) In view of the relatively high incidence of AIDS among male homosexuals and bisexuals, it is necessary to develop a knowledge of their life-style. The male homosexual patients are usually willing teachers — it is essential that the nurse be receptive to information they give. Peers will help clarify obscure aspects.

(3) In order to avoid judging others, it is extremely useful for the nurse to study his or her own sexuality. This is best done through discussion with close friends, sexual partners and, in some instances, peers on the ward.

(4) In order to develop sensitivity towards dying patients, it is worth learning self-awareness and knowing one's own attitudes to death as well as developing tools for use with other people. Workshops for this purpose are available (see Chapter 11).

Stress and Powerlessness

Levels of stress are high for nurses caring for AIDS patients. The number of decisions and the importance of decisions, especially with regard to psychological care, are increased beyond the levels normally found on general wards. These forms of stress can easily be controlled by providing enough nurses and ensuring that they rapidly develop the new skills required. However, it is the nature of institutional and economic response that a gap develops between a rapid growth in need (the number of AIDS sufferers doubling every 8 months) and the actual provision of adequate resources. This often gives rise to a sense of powerlessness.

There are four problems that are not so easily dealt with by increasing resources.

(1) Because many of the male homosexual patients continue to compartmentalise their lives, they may wish some people to know and others not to know their diagnosis, etc. In order to function properly, the nurse has to remember and record precisely who is who and what they know. Mistakes are both unethical and costly in terms of care.

(2) The nurse becomes closely involved with the patient, his or her lover, the parental family and friends. The nurse shares in the knowledge of their domestic details and also shares in the unrelenting swing between hope and despair. This is a particular form of emotional stress common to high-dependency nursing areas that have mortality rates.

(3) The nurse is continually subjecting herself to risks of becoming seropositive (through inoculation of patient blood, and exposure to secretions) or contracting other serious disease (CMV). The risks are *very small indeed*, but her exposure is large and the possible consequences are catastrophic. She depends on both her and her colleagues' judgement and good technique.

(4) The nurse fulfils a variety of roles in society. She or he is daughter or son, girl-friend or boy-friend, wife or husband to other men and women. These men and women, especially under powerful influence of the media, often exert pressure on their loved ones not to nurse this group of patients. This is the source of inevitable emotional conflict for the nurse. In addition, the nurse is worried that the exposure may result in her unknowingly transmitting the virus to other members of her family.

Support

The stresses and powerlessness as well as practical but recurring problems require identifying, expressing and solving where possible. The group capable of doing this is a nursing or caring team support group. It needs to meet regularly; it must not be controlled by hierarchical figures; and it may need a facilitator (a person versed in group dynamics) with no vested interests. The usual difficulty is that of obtaining a good attendance, owing to commitment to 24 h care and the need to get away when off duty. The nurse manager must provide opportunity in terms of time and staffing; given this opportunity, despite the difficulties, it is usual for nurses to form the group as they perceive the need. The nurse manager should also ensure that any financial benefits allowable are provided — for example, the Sexually Transmitted Disease lead (4% of salary) in the UK.

Nurse Manager

The number of AIDS sufferers in the UK is doubling every 8 months. Many nurse managers are being asked to give estimates of nursing and other resources required in their area of responsibility.

Staffing

The following is a check-list of the essential information.

(1) Projection of number of AIDS, ARC and PGL patients.

(2) Define your brief exactly. Is your brief global? Are you expected to consider all requirements of these patients or simply those functions that you are responsible for (e.g. intensive care, ward, operating theatres, endoscopy unit, out-patients and community care)? Many ancillary services will be affected — e.g. portering, transport, domestics.

(3) Bed management policy with regard to: (a) all patients; (b) AIDS + ARC patients; (c) PGL patients (e.g. requiring lymph node biopsy); (d) HTLV-III-positive (e.g. to be nursed in single rooms or open wards).

(4) Current medical practice in treatment of opportunist infections (e.g. mean length of stay of patients suffering from *Pneumocystis carinii* pneumonia); use of trial drugs and degree of striving for life — use of intensive care.

(5) Space available (e.g. number of beds — whether on open ward or in single rooms).

(6) On the basis of the above, predict the bed occupancy (of each facility) by (a) all patients; (b) acutely ill AIDS + ARC patients; (c) AIDS + ARC patients who require investigation or convalescence; (d) HTLV-III-positive and PGL patients requiring treatment of an unrelated disorder.

If information is not available, discuss all possible outcomes with as many involved colleagues as possible and make assumptions. If necessary, draw up two different proposals based on two different groups of assumptions. Always state very precisely the assumptions made, so that no misunderstanding can arise.

If a system for calculating nursing establishments, applicable to a large range of patient dependency, is already in use in your institution, then use this recognised method. If no such system exists and if there is already a little experience gained in caring for AIDS sufferers, a modified version of the Telford Consultative Approach (see References and Bibliography) is a useful and acceptable tool. If there is no previous experience of nursing AIDS sufferers, then visit an institution with similar facilities, create models of patients and use these in a modified Telford Consultative Approach with the staff who are to care for the patients. See Appendix 2 for an example.

EQUIPMENT

Remember to consider all equipment that is: (a) directly the concern of the nurse (e.g. commodes/toilets — one for each patient — and intravenous pumps — increased usage and need for portability); (b) indirectly the concern of the nurse (e.g. proctoscopes and sigmoidoscopes should be disposable wherever possible, because recycling is relatively dangerous for nursing and ancillary staff). Request a capital sum to be made available for a given list of possible equipment needs. It is cheaper and more efficient not to commit oneself too far ahead.

MANAGEMENT OF THE AIDS SUFFERER IN THE COMMUNITY – SOME OBSERVATIONS AND PROPOSALS

No systematic approach to care of this group at home exists in the UK at present. The vast majority of AIDS sufferers who return home after admission to hospital look to their own or charitable resources for continuing care. The focus of continuing advice and technical care simply switches back to the sexually transmitted disease (STD) clinic or out-patients' department (OPD). The community nurse occasionally takes on a practical nursing role at home, but only when the GP is involved. Patients often do not wish the hospital consultant to refer them to their GP, and there is some general acceptance of this state of affairs by GPs. In addition, community nurses do not provide a hospice service.

The San Francisco General Hospital has developed a ward-based hospice nursing service. The hospice nurses visit the patients and provide counselling support and organise physical care (which is also carried out by nursing aides/volunteers*). They work in the ward, updating themselves and teaching patients and other nurses, as well as providing high levels of continuity for the patient moving from out-patients' to ward and thence to home and out-patients' again. They visit patients on other wards when they are admitted for investigations and surgery, and they also teach nurses on these wards. The Macmillan teams in this country have already established the approach to a similar group of patients (dying cancer patients).

In those hospitals that provide an AIDS in-patients' service for a health district, it is essential that in future hospice nurses be included as part of the care team and be allowed to give both practical nursing care and expert advice to all AIDS patients in the district. They must move from clinic to ward to home as the needs of the AIDS sufferer dictates. The OPD/STD clinic doctor (an AIDS specialist) should be the prescriber with whom the hospice nurse works, thus ensuring team continuity.

It is by these means that the goal of dying with dignity at home may be achieved.

---

*The Terrence Higgins Trust provides a 'Buddy Volunteer Service' in England.

APPENDIX 1: EXAMPLE OF ASEPTIC PROCEDURES USED FOR TOTAL PARENTERAL NUTRITION THERAPY

Changing Bag for Parenteral Feeding Lines (Subclavian Position)

Prepare patient.

Nurse	*Assistant (2nd Nurse)*
(1) Both nurses and patient put on face mask.	
(2) Wash hands thoroughly.	Take trolley to bedside. Alcowipe top of trolley and drop procedure pack on top. Place bag on clip on side of trolley.
(3)	Expose patient's chest area.
(4) Take gloves and put them on.	Open gloves.
(5) Open pack and prepare.	Pour iodine into gallipot. Open non-adherent dressing and shield onto sterile field.
(6)	Remove old adhesive tape and old shield and non-adherent dressing. Hold giving set away from patient's skin. Be careful not to handle connection area.
(7) Clean skin with Betadine and place sterile towels under connection.	
(8)	Spray connection and tubing with alcohol, making sure Luer Lock is sprayed thoroughly. Turn off giving set and pass mosquito forceps ready for use.
(9) Clamp extension tube. Hold Luer Lock in sterile gauze, wipe connection with Betadine thoroughly. Unscrew connection and discard old giving set. Hold remaining Luer Lock for 2nd nurse to spray.	Spray connection inside and outside with alcohol.
(10) Take new giving set, holding it with sterile gauze, and remove sterile cap. Wipe connection with Betadine and hold in position ready for 2nd nurse to spray.	Spray connection thoroughly with alcohol.
(11) Connect new giving set and remove clamp.	
(12) Observe extension tubing for air.	

(13) Apply shield. Remove sterile
       towels. Apply non-adherent
       dressing to connection and place
       adhesive tape along tubing to
       cover connection area.
(14) Remove mask from patient.   Regulate drip. Leave patient comfort-
       Tidy trolley, clean and put away.   able.

APPENDIX 2: NURSING REQUIREMENTS FOR NURSING SEVERELY ILL AIDS AND ARC PATIENTS CARED FOR IN FOURTEEN-BED SINGLE-ROOM ISOLATION WARD

Assumptions

(1) A fixed eight-bed admission policy will be in successful operation.

(2) The mean number of beds occupied by this group of patients would be 8.

(3) The remaining patients will be mainly seriously ill infectious disease patients.

(4) PGL patients requiring lymph node biopsy but otherwise fairly well will be cared for by the surgeon concerned in his own ward bed.

(5) The mean bed occupancy of the ward will be 13.

The staffing of the ward was considered as a whole. It is not acceptable to consider the 8 AIDS patients as a separate entity, because distortions in estimates of staffing needs would result.

Method

Models of 8 AIDS patients and ARC (AIDS-related complex) patients were described and discussed in a group consisting of Staff Nurse, Sister, Senior Nurse and Assistant Director of Nursing Services. A mix of patients needs and problems was based on our experience over the past 18 months. In addition, it was assumed that there would normally be 5 of the higher-dependency infectious disease patients on the ward at the same time. A modified Telford Consultative Approach was utilised to estimate the establishment required.

Conclusion

$7\frac{1}{2}$ h shifts to be utilised with the following numbers of staff: 6 early shift; 5 late shift; 4 night shift. The required establishment for these levels of staffing would be 27.8 whole-time equivalents (WTE) utilising a supplement of 21% for annual leave, study leave and sickness. However, a 7.5% addition is required for extensive study leave, mainly to learn and strengthen counselling skills. The final total required is 30 WTE.

REFERENCES AND BIBLIOGRAPHY

Communicable Disease Report. PHLS Communicable Disease Surveillance Centre, 61 Colindale Avenue, London NW9

Hector, W. and Whitfield, S. (1982). *Nursing Care for the Dying Patient and Family*. London, Heinemann

Kubler-Ross, E. (1970). *On Death and Dying*. London, Tavistock

Morbidity and Mortality Weekly Report (Collection June 1981 through January 1985). Atlanta, Georgia, Centres for Disease Control

Morrison, M. L. (1980). *Respiratory Intensive Care Nursing from Beth Israel Hospital, Boston*. Boston, Little Brown

O'Brien, D. and Alexander, S. (Eds.) (1985). *High Dependency Nursing Care*. Edinburgh, Churchill Livingstone

Telford Consultative Approach (1983). *Determining Nursing Establishments*. Birmingham, England

WORKSHOPS

AIDS Workshop: David Miller, St Mary's Hospital, Praed Street, London W2

Life, Death and Transition: E. Kubler-Ross, Shanti Nilaya (England), PO Box 212, London NW8

CRUSE Counselling Workshops and Support Groups: C. Spence, Lifestory Counselling Centre, 178 Lancaster Road, London W11

7

Psychology, AIDS, ARC and PGL

David Miller

INTRODUCTION

In the context of the psychological issues generated by AIDS, the counsellor or therapist is rather like the conductor of an orchestra in which the players are the patient, the lover, family, friends, employers and the hospital staff. They must co-ordinate relevant information from these varied sources, they must initiate and maintain an informed understanding with all those involved, and they need to keep an eye on all subsequent developments, altering the emphasis of intervention as circumstances change. Some degree of discord seems inevitable, but with preparation, flexibility and understanding this may be kept to a minimum, and much benefit may be derived for the patient.

It must be said that counselling people with AIDS is not a suitable task for everyone, and not all patients want or need advice. Some patients want to know simply what their condition involves, the prognosis, and ways of reducing their risk of further infection and infectivity to others. Where psychological counselling is appropriate, it is in many respects more demanding than counselling with other conditions. Many people with AIDS are terminally ill, and for this reason alone intervention requires reliability, consistency and continuity.

The requirement for sensitivity and a non-judgemental approach towards homosexuality (where patients are homosexual) is obvious. Counsellors should preferably have previous experience with psychological management, but this is not as important as common-sense and an awareness of one's own limits in dealing with the problems of others. However, it is *vital* to have a clear understanding of the syndrome and its associated medical effects.

INFORMING THE PATIENT OF THE DIAGNOSIS

When the patient is being informed of the diagnosis, straight talking is essential. Giving such information is never easy, and some doctors may feel that gentle hinting or not giving the full picture is somehow more palatable for the patient, but this is rarely the case. It is clear from clinical reports and discussion with patients that avoidance or dilution of the facts of their diagnosis results in a more difficult adjustment for them, and adds resentment and a loss of confidence to their subsequent dealings with health professionals.

Many of the patients receiving a diagnosis of AIDS, AIDS-related complex (ARC) or persistent generalised lymphadenopathy (PGL) will have been ill for some time, and will have anticipated their doctor's statement, particularly after the widespread media attention the syndrome has received. For these persons, diagnosis may bring a kind of 'relief' from the uncertainty of their pre-diagnosis condition – they know at last what they are up against. The uncertainty is then focused on the future and on methods of survival. For others, the appearance and confirmation of diagnostic signs may come quite unexpectedly, possibly provoking the reactions frequently reported in cancer patients (Dilley *et al.*, 1985) and other terminally ill groups (Morin *et al.*, 1984). This is because diagnoses of AIDS, ARC or PGL are typically viewed by the patient as terminal, irrespective of the extent of the associated infections or disorders.

Irrespective of the degree to which the patient is prepared for the news, it involves some degree of shock which may well create a 'numbness' or 'stunned' withdrawal, during which explanations by the informing doctor are not fully registered. This is particularly so where a patient has a catastrophic shock reaction involving verbal anger, disbelief, crying, physical agitation and fear. This raises two points. First, the informing doctor should not take angry verbal responses personally, as they are an expected part of a shock reaction. Second, whether or not patients become unreceptive because of their immediate emotional reaction, staff concerned should encourage them to attend for a further appointment in the *near* future (7–14 days), perhaps with their lover or a close friend or family member, having written down questions they will inevitably want answered at that later time.

IMPLICATIONS OF DIAGNOSIS

A diagnosis of AIDS has profound implications for the patient. The prediction of death that most make in conjunction with diagnosis, the chilling realisation that no cure yet exists and that friends and others are dying of AIDS, and the widely unsympathetic response of the public to affected homosexuals, generates a sense of entrapment for most patients, especially in the first few months following the news. Some of those affected have described AIDS, ARC or PGL as a prison from which there is no escape. Understandably, many have talked of experiencing a 'revolution' in their life since they became aware of their condition. Accordingly, the effect of diagnosis is felt in many important ways.

Personal Control

Persons with AIDS feel that they have a much reduced control over their life and the options that are now available to them. They feel they are no longer a 'free agent', and that every activity they undertake is predicated on their disease and the prospect of illness and death. The current absence of a cure for AIDS and HTLV-III infection emphasises their powerlessness over the syndrome, and a sense of helplessness can frequently arise and inhibit possible constructive moves in the future.

Because AIDS is still incurable and treatments for subsequent infections and sarcomas remain largely experimental, patients undergo intensive 'medicalisation' after diagnosis. Their post-diagnostic lives are initially centred around the hospital and the medical staff, and social, domestic and work schedules are greatly interrupted to allow this. Thus, many patients come to feel that they have become 'guinea-pigs', and that their personal identity and control is lost behind the testing, probing, observation and medication that the relative novelty of their illness generates. Some are very pleased to co-operate with such intensive scrutiny, while others become distressed at what they may eventually regard as intrusive experimentation.

Again, the need for a full explanation from staff about the reasoning behind such treatment activity can help the patient's adjustment to this change of emphasis in routine (particularly where infections are not in themselves disruptive). A consistent feature of patient reactions to diagnosis is the appreciation gained from frank discussion with staff about their situation and future. It helps greatly to reduce the strain of medicalisation felt by both the patient and the lover or family, and enables the circumstances to be put into a concrete perspective. Any activity that helps to reduce uncertainty and a feeling of loss of control in the patient (even where decline is apparent) promotes realistic adjustment and effective rapport with staff.

Self-esteem

AIDS is a severely stigmatising illness. It is not a 'glamorous' disease, nor is it one that excites public sympathy. On the contrary, it is usually received in lay circles with fear and avoidance. Evidence for this is reported by patients who have experienced 'shunning' by friends, colleagues, employees and associates. For many, such a public response (and/or the anticipation of it) generates a feeling of being unclean or dirty. Many patients suggest that they have become a 'social leper' and will avoid discussing their diagnosis with others for fear of the anticipated response occurring. Such worries emphasise the need for the therapist or practitioner to maintain a non-judgemental attitude towards the patient and his sexual history.

In this context, unresolved conflicts over the patients' homosexuality are likely to emerge, particularly where the process of 'coming out' has been associated with a family trauma such as divorce or parental non-acceptance. Many homosexuals remain uneasy about their sexuality, some managing their guilt or anxiety mainly by periodic, anonymous sex with others, or by staying in 'the closet'. For such patients, the diagnosis offers further 'evidence' of their 'wrong-doing', and much self-recrimination and personal blame can result.

Self-esteem is further affected in cases where Kaposi's sarcomas, weight loss and infections cause physical, particularly facial, disfigurement. A number of patients with facial symptoms report withdrawing from social and work situations because they feel too self-conscious or unattractive. Of course, a proliferation of, for example, sarcomas to facial and scalp areas often heralds a quickening of the patient's physical decline, recognition of which compounds the sense of helplessness.

Social Implications

As mentioned above, many affected homosexuals choose to keep their diagnosis to themselves, and while this may largely be due to a fear of 'discovery' and of the reaction of others, it is also due often to a fear of infecting those close to them. Patients will frequently be as ignorant of the syndrome as the public at large, and they require detailed information concerning the level of risk they present to others, in the home, at work, socially and sexually.

Some of the patients seen will be relatively isolated socially. The homosexual 'community' comprises many sub-groups; and if the patient has not been a part of an established social circle, has irregular employment or has personality problems that prevent the establishment of lasting relationships or friendships, the advent of diagnosis emphasises his loneliness and isolation. Indeed, for some, sexual activity may have been their only means of making social contact, and so their illness effectively cuts them off from future contact. For others, perhaps in the context of established relationships, the impact of their diagnosis on the lover may be a paramount concern. For instance, they may worry that the lover will 'desert' them, leaving them to die alone, or that they have passed the virus on to their loved one.

The physical impact of diagnosis on social activity varies with the diagnostic symptoms, of course, and where *Pneumocystis carinii* pneumonia and other infections are problematic, fatigue and lethargy together with the effects of anxiety may result in an inability to socialise on a previously enjoyed scale. In such circumstances, it may be necessary to counsel the lover about the partner's restricted abilities, so that undue resentment and relationship strain do not complicate the picture.

Occupational Disruption

The presenting patient may be very ill and unable to keep working for some time after diagnosis. The question then frequently becomes one of what to tell employers and colleagues. In view of recent media coverage of the syndrome, many work colleagues aware of the patient's sexuality may have jumped to conclusions about the patient's condition. In other cases, no one else may suspect the diagnosis, leaving the patient with the option of providing information. The universal fear is that employers' knowledge of the illness will result in dismissal, and this, unfortunately, has been common. In other cases, patients have reported that union representatives have been similarly reluctant to fight for their consideration, which has resulted in the AIDS patient losing job or career and facing considerable financial hardship.

It is therefore understandable that the patient may be reluctant to make the full facts of his condition known. Many have chosen to leave work, giving their employers a more 'acceptable' diagnosis as the reason − e.g. 'terminal cancer', 'leukaemia', or 'tuberculosis'. Those who choose to stay at work have described similarly incapacitating conditions requiring frequent medical intervention, and have kept working until the illness has made this impracticable. In order to decide which option is most appropriate, much consideration needs to be given to the company's previous experience of the syndrome, the nature of the work the patient is required to do, the amount of travelling involved, and so on. Telling the full truth of diagnosis may have clearly disastrous career and financial implications, although it is worth bearing in mind that the anxiety and stress associated with not telling the whole story may be detrimental to the patient's general adjustment after diagnosis. It is also clear that what information is given by doctors and patients to employers must be agreed upon beforehand, to minimise any risk of unnecessary career loss. As with many other psychological disorders, the routine and distraction of regular work (where health permits) helps to provide relief from the anxiety and morbid obsession with illness and death that characterises adjustment to diagnosis in many cases.

Emotional Implications

Emotional reactions to the shock of diagnosis have already been discussed. However the emotional consequences of diagnosis do not stop there. An underlying feature of the period following diagnosis, reported by many patients, is that of unremitting anxiety. This may be due to a number of factors, many of which reflect the concerns being currently addressed. Particular sources of anxiety are listed in Table 7.1.

A common and worrying feature of anxiety, particularly at high levels, is the range of symptoms involving the autonomic nervous system (ANS). For those with PGL and ARC, in particular, the ANS effects, such as diarrhoea, nausea, resultant weight loss, sweating, shaking, visual disturbances, muscle pains, skin rashes and lethargy, are frequently interpreted as being signs of AIDS, and resulting worries about this tend to make the symptoms worse, possibly leading to acute anxiety (panic) attacks. For those with AIDS, such symptoms are often interpreted as indications of a decline in their physical status, resulting in further distress.

Table 7.1   Some emotional implications of AIDS and PGL diagnosis

Shock:
   of diagnosis and possible death; uncertainty
Anxiety:
   uncertain prognosis and course of illness
   effects of medication and treatment
   status of lover, and lover's ability to cope
   reactions of others (family, friends, lover, colleagues, employers, etc.)
   loss of cognitive, physical, social and occupational abilities
   risk of infection from and to others
Depression:
   helpless to change circumstances
   virus in control of life
   reduced quality of life in all spheres
   gloomy, possibly painful, uncomfortable and disfiguring, future
   self-blame and recriminations for past 'indiscretions'
   reduced social and sexual acceptability, and isolation
Anger:
   over past high-risk life-style and activities
   over inability to overcome the virus
   over new and involuntary life-style restrictions
Guilt:
   being homosexual
   'confirmed' unacceptability of homosexuality via illness
Obsessions:
   relentless searching for explanations
   relentless searching for new diagnostic evidence on his own body
   inevitability of decline and death
   faddism over health and diets

A further common clinical observation concerns the emotional strain of alternating fears and hopes. The patient may awake one morning feeling cheerful and optimistic for the future only to 'crash' later into a trough of despair as trivial day-to-day circumstances drain his stamina and hopes for recovery. Such a pattern undermines the patient's confidence that things may improve or that a cure will one day be found, and depression may quickly result after a succession of short-lived pleasures.

Depression leads to its own difficulties, particularly where it results in a loss of motivation to 'fight' for the future or to comply with treatment regimens that hold promise for the patient. A loss of interest in previously rewarding activities (at home and work) is also characteristic, and can contribute to a general functional decline and withdrawal. Depression has, in one study, been found to be the most typical psychological problem in AIDS patients (Dilley *et al.*, 1985), and appears to result from real or imagined isolation following diagnosis, uncertainty about the future, and sadness at the loss of health, income, employability and future relationships. It has been observed to follow closely from the patient's perception of AIDS being a form of punishment for his homosexuality.

Much concern by the patient for the fate of the lover is, understandably, in evidence. The lover in many ways has a multiple burden, in so far as he — indirectly, at least — suffers the involuntary constraints of the physical and emotional effects of AIDS diagnosis (reduced social and sexual options, financial pressures, etc.), and must then assume the role of full-time domestic nurse, counsellor and care-taker, while acting often as middle-man in the discussions between the patient, the hospital, family and friends. For some relationships, the strain will eventually prove too much, and further distress is created by arguments and even separation. In cases where neurological damage results in a severe change of personality and ability in the patient, lovers have been 'given permission' to leave the relationship as domestic management becomes resentful and fraught, and the patient's unreliability and insufficiency threatens the physical and emotional safety of both.

Further emotional implications may be seen in the reactions of families and colleagues in whom the occasion of AIDS highlights a fundamental opposition to homosexuality. Diagnosis may be held up as a confirmation of the 'evil' that homosexuality embodies, and their subsequent dealings with the patient and his life-style become hostile and resentful. On the other hand, diagnosis can actually bring previously fragile family relationships to a sounder, more secure and understanding footing, much to the surprise and pleasure of the patient, who may have worried greatly about family reactions.

Sexual Implications

AIDS has highlighted the widespread ignorance in empirical and medical circles about homosexuality in general, and homosexual sexual activity in particular (Green and Miller, 1985). However, information from patients has indicated two main consequences for the sexuality of gay men.

First, diagnosis creates *functional* disturbances, most commonly an initial loss of libido and/or erectile dysfunction, together with the behavioural restrictions following from suggested guidelines for safer sex (see Chapter 10).

Second, AIDS creates *conceptual* disturbances for the patient, which can be very wide-ranging. It must be appreciated that, for many homosexuals, sexual activity is of central importance. While a great number of gay men lead relatively conventional sexual lives that appear to mirror the experiences of most heterosexuals, many others regard sexual activity as a means of homosexual affirmation; a continuing expression of their sexual identity in the face of perceived widespread social oppression and distaste. This is not to say that, for such men, sex necessarily represents a continuous and delicious banquet — many report that a high level of casual sex results in emotional emptiness or dissatisfaction, but they remain involved in such activity in order to maintain some social contact, or to find a stable partner with whom they can 'settle down'. Nevertheless, gay clubs and pubs do allow an opportunity to mix without the risk of social hostility or intolerance.

AIDS thus brings a critical interruption to the gay life-style. There is a loss of the hard-won homosexual identity and group affirmation resulting from the loss of 'easy' sexual activity, and this may well explain why a few patients remain sexually active despite the risks to themselves and others. There is also the under-mining of homosexuality as an increasingly acceptable social category. Any increased tolerance of homosexuality in society which may have been established in the pre-AIDS era has now been lost because of the high association of homo-sexuality with the disease.

This has led, in a number of cases, to high levels of guilt concerning gay sexuality and sexual practices, with the patient attempting to bargain his way out of the illness by vowing to 'go straight' and become heterosexual (while also denouncing all homosexuality). Many patients blame themselves for their ill-ness, regarding it as some form of punishment for being homosexual, and in such cases depression is frequently a consequence.

Cognitive and Neurological Implications

There are predictable cognitive effects following from the anxiety and depression that accompany diagnosis and the strains of adjustment to AIDS. These include higher levels of distractability, memory impairment, poor concentration, im-paired orientation and general confusion. However, it is clear that many frank neurological features associated with central nervous system (CNS) diseases may also emerge to complicate management. Active agents in the appearance of such disturbances include infections such as toxoplasmosis, cytomegalovirus, and cryptococcal and other menengitides (responsible for, for example, subacute encephalitis, visual disturbances and blindness, etc.), neoplasms (including CNS Kaposi's sarcoma and immunoblastic lymphomas), and cerebrovascular disease (Snider *et al.*, 1983). Some acute organic mental disorders, such as delirium, may be caused by disorders secondary to physical diseases in AIDS — for example, hypoxaemia secondary to *Pneumocystis carinii* pneumonia, and metabolic im-balance secondary to diarrhoea, sepsis and post-ictal conditions (Wolcott, 1984).

Behavioural effects of CNS disorders in AIDS are seen in *affective disturbances* producing inappropriate (emotional) responses to crises, or to medical, social and domestic events; *personality disorders* resulting in unpredictable and awkward character changes; *dementia-like syndromes* involving disturbances in memory, concentration, orientation, speech defects and increasing cognitive unreliability; and states of *delirium* (see Chapter 1).

A problem with CNS involvement is that resulting behavioural changes can be very insidious, and the practitioner needs to be on guard for the possibility of neurological impairment wherever psychological or psychiatric symptoms appear. One recent survey found that 31% (50/160) of patients had neurological disease prior to death from AIDS (Snider *et al.*, 1983). It is also important to note that the existence of neurological problems does not preclude psychological difficulties in patients.

Other Implications

It is clear that uncertainty is a central feature for the person with AIDS, ARC or PGL. For those with AIDS, the uncertainty concerns the course of the syndrome, the prognosis (in the short and long term), the efficacy of medical treatments, and issues such as the effects on the lover and the family. For those with ARC PGL, uncertainty concerns the prospect of 'advancing' into AIDS. In this context, anxiety and preoccupation with illness can be considerable, in some cases developing into a clinical obsessive-compulsive syndrome. With this syndrome, the patient is preoccupied with involuntary and distressing thoughts and/or mental images of AIDS infection, and with the consequences of developing AIDS. The patient will recognise periodically that such preoccupations are out of proportion to the known facts about the illness, and may be receptive to reasoned counselling for brief periods, but the thoughts inevitably return. In many cases, anxiety produced by such thoughts will compel the patient to check his body for indications or signs of infection. In time, checking can become a major disruption, occupying many hours daily as resistance to the thoughts crumbles.

TREATMENT

The therapist's treatment intervention essentially involves (a) putting the illness in a factual, realistic perspective; (b) structuring the issues the patient is required to face so that his responses to the disease are relevant and effective, not vague and floundering. Both aspects emphasise the necessity of restoring the patient's perceived self-control over the syndrome.

Managing the Early Stages

Typically, the newly diagnosed AIDS patient will receive an initial period of hospitalisation in order to complete diagnostic procedures, and/or to provide treatment for presenting infections. This period may vary, according to the severity of symptoms, from a few days to a few weeks. (A small number of patients who are first diagnosed during the later stages of the syndrome may die during their first admission.) This means that initial contact with the patient is usually made shortly after admission, and it is desirable that the counsellor should be introduced to the patient during this early stage, in order to establish his or her role as part of the 'team'. Later introductions to 'the psychologist' or 'the counsellor' are sometimes met with some resistance from patients because they fear that others must think they are crazy!

The main aim of this early intervention is to assist the patient in coming to terms with his diagnosis, both intellectually and emotionally (Miller and Green, 1985). The shock of diagnosis naturally raises questions from the patient, which need to be answered in a straightforward, frank way. Much discussion inevitably centres on the prognosis. Where possible, the staff should avoid attempting to give a prognosis, particularly estimates of time left to live. Such estimates could well be quite wrong, and they tend to take hope away. Patients who have been told they will be dead in so many months or years will usually accept this information, and the incentive to fight for life, or even a better quality of life remaining, can be destroyed by the apparent certainty of the medical authority. Dwelling on the statistics of mortality is similarly unhelpful, and can lead to helplessness and pessimism. General statistics are not relevant to individual cases, and although many patients will be aware of the bleak prognoses associated with particular illnesses, the emphasis should be more on prospects for maintenance and recovery. Replies should be honest and constructive, not destructive. In these circumstances no one can honestly say when a patient will die, and the job of the staff is to promote health — not to pass death sentences!

Having said that, it is necessary for many people to discuss the possibility of their dying in order to get the syndrome into perspective and to decide how to cope with 'loose ends'. However, the decision to discuss such topics should be the patient's, and they need to be faced without fear or embarrassment on the part of the therapist. Again, it is not necessary to add estimates of mortality to such talks, as constructive discussion may well provide an initial spur to mobilise the patient's resources in the coming fight for life against the virus.

Where questions cannot be answered for the patient, he should be given an explanation of why they cannot be answered. The requirement for close liaison between the counsellor and the physician in charge in such circumstances is obvious.

It is important at this stage to move on to a full assessment of how the patient is reacting to diagnosis. Many reactions have already been discussed above, and the patient needs to be allowed to talk at some length about these. The counsellor can then probe gently for signs of particular difficulty, which can then be followed up at later sessions. This is also a good time to introduce the matters of infection control, domestic management and general risk-reduction, perhaps with the lover or family member present. The patient may wish to be reassured about measures he can take to maintain sexual relations with the lover at this time.

Those who have been diagnosed as being HTLV-III-positive with ARC or PGL will frequently respond with high levels of anxiety and, sometimes, depression, particularly because they are left with a distressing 'waiting game' as to the eventual direction their virus infection will lead them. The information may serve as a catalyst (as with newly diagnosed AIDS patients) for the ventilation of previously unmentioned and troubling emotional issues within stable relationships, and the counsellor must therefore be alert for potentially destructive themes arising in this manner. Many react to diagnosis by making a complete re-evaluation of their lives and activities, but the considerable uncertainty remains ever-present no matter what they or the therapist or counsellor can do.

In view of this situation, the ventilation and unforced discussion encouraged with AIDS patients may be applied to ARC and PGL patients as well, in order to allow an assessment of those patient qualities which may be used to provide a basis for an effective and relevant coping response. With all groups, it is necessary to assure the patient that he has an 'open door' to the counsellor, so he or his lover can ring for advice as required between sessions.

One final point at this stage: the patient should be urged to take great care over who else is told about the diagnosis at this time. For instance, employers' and family members' reactions must be carefully assessed and prepared for with the counsellor first.

Managing the Process of Adjustment to Diagnosis

After the initial stage of ventilation, answering immediate questions and providing basic information, the process of adjustment is faced. Although adjustments may be necessary in many areas (see under 'Implications of Diagnosis', above), the promotion of self-control requires that the patient be helped to achieve a position from which he can make necessary changes for himself. In order to allow this, counselling intervention typically involves procedures for the management of anxiety, depression and obsessive (compulsive) disorders, together with the application of appropriate information and social facilities (e.g. social worker, community workers) that make effective management possible after diagnosis. A schematic structure for counselling intervention is presented in Figure 7.1.

In order to determine the impact of anxiety, depression, etc., on the adjustment of the patient, it is helpful to ask him how he has been affected by the diagnosis – i.e. how the diagnosis has made problems for him. This can be done by a form of problem analysis in which the problems are set alongside hypotheses, solutions, assets and deficits which the patient may bring to the problem setting (see Chapter 8). In performing such a 'problem breakdown', the most realistic solutions can be found. An example of the format employed is given in Table 7.2. This structured approach to post-diagnostic difficulties is pragmatic and efficient, and can be employed again whenever problems arise, for all those personally involved with the patient. Solutions arising may range from putting legal and financial affairs in order (e.g. making a will, settling tax issues) to 'making the peace' with family or friends so that the patient is no longer unnecessarily burdened or alienated by past events. Naturally, the plans made by the patient must take realistic account of his physical state and the likely course of the syndrome.

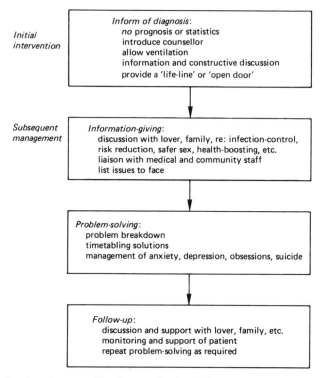

Initial intervention

Inform of diagnosis:
no prognosis or statistics
introduce counsellor
allow ventilation
information and constructive discussion
provide a 'life-line' or 'open door'

Subsequent management

Information-giving:
discussion with lover, family, re: infection-control, risk reduction, safer sex, health-boosting, etc.
liaison with medical and community staff
list issues to face

Problem-solving:
problem breakdown
timetabling solutions
management of anxiety, depression, obsessions, suicide

Follow-up:
discussion and support with lover, family, etc.
monitoring and support of patient
repeat problem-solving as required

Figure 7.1 Structure for counselling intervention in AIDS, ARC and PGL

Managing Anxiety

It is important to recognise that anxiety, like depression, is a *normal* human response to life-threatening illness, and it is therefore to be expected. In this context, however, anxiety appears to be more severe and of a longer duration, and as it seems clear that prolonged anxiety is itself immunosuppressive (Coates *et al.*, 1984), the need for effective intervention is paramount. Some people might argue that such effort is wasteful, as the external uncertainty prompting anxiety, especially for ARC PGL patients, can never be overcome. However, despite this, much can be done to reduce inner distress, and strategies arising from problem breakdowns together with anxiety management techniques have had considerable clinical benefits in a large number of cases (Miller and Green, 1985). Anxiety management can also be of use for AIDS, ARC and PGL patients, because anxiety symptoms (such as sweating, muscle pains, fatigue, etc.) are frequently interpreted as indications of declining physical health, and thus add considerably to the distress of the patient and his domestic unit (cf. Miller *et al.*, 1985). The symptoms and diagnosis of anxiety are fully covered in Chapter 8.

The course of intervention for anxiety is as follows.

(1) Ask the patient about the reasons for his anxiety (ventilation).
(2) Restate known information about his illness, about what constructive

Table 7.2 Patient problem analysis

Problem	Links and hypotheses	Possible solutions	Patient difficulties	Patient assets	Priorities
Depressed mood, poor sleep, withdrawn	Depression	Depression management	Doesn't like medication	Motivated to change	1
Cannot inform parents	Anxious about their reaction (Dad very anti-gay)	Tell selected relatives; coach and practice telling	Father very anti-gay	Close to sister, who is close to father	3
Few outside social contacts	Social isolation; few opportunities	Seek existing friends; join clubs, groups	Friends become sexual partners	Wide interests; happy with celibacy; socially skilled	4
Dizzy, nausea, palpitations, sweating	Anxiety	Anxiety management	Difficulty in separating anxiety from AIDS symptoms	Intelligent and receptive to information	2
Exlusively anal and oral–anal	Habit	Modify sex behaviour; mutual masturbation?	None	Likes mutual masturbation; happy with celibacy	6
Offered sex frequently	Well known in gay clubs and pubs	Socialise elsewhere	None	Assertive and socially skilled	5

moves are being made to help him medically and about methods of personal risk reduction and health boosting.

(3) Explain how anxiety works, why it can lead to panic attacks, and why he feels the symptoms the way he does.

(4) Provide liaison between relevant hospital departments so that necessary information can be obtained if the patient has been worrying over delays, etc.

(5) Provide relaxation training to reduce topical and baseline autonomic arousal, and as a self-control strategy for physical relief.

(6) Encourage the planning of distracting and enjoyable activities in order to provide relief from anxiety and stimulate positive attitudes towards the circumstances.

(7) Use cognitive aids, such as lists of 'fact statements' about anxiety, personal strengths, positive achievements, etc., to stimulate motivation and positive thinking. Also, rational discussion can help to undermine negative, anxiety-producing thinking.

(8) Encourage socialisation where appropriate, perhaps through support or interest groups.

(9) Anxiolytic medication can be useful in some cases, for *short* periods. Dependence should be avoided, and side-effects may outweigh possible benefits. In cases of extreme anxiety, anxiolytics can be used as a short-term aid to sleep.

In most cases, anxiety seems to follow a 'roller-coaster' pattern, where periods of acute anxiety will suddenly give way to periods of relative calm. Onset of acute anxiety tends to be associated often with the appearance of new media headlines about AIDS, even after other adjustments have been successfully made. The appearance of repeated or new infections and symptoms also triggers renewed bouts of anxiety, and the suggestions made may need to be repeated.

Managing Depression

The symptoms and diagnosis of depression are covered in Chapter 8 and will not be repeated here. However, it is worth stating that, like anxiety, depression must be recognised as an expected response to diagnosis and the uncertainty that accompanies it. A difficulty frequently faced is the way in which symptoms of anxiety and depression may overlap, making clear diagnosis difficult. This lack of clarity is made worse when the possibility of neurological impairment leading to some of the common symptom patterns exists, as it often does in this context (see above). If doubt exists as to the cause of presenting psychosomatic symptoms, exclude the possibility of more serious disorders by working backwards through diagnostic protocols. For example, in order to assess whether the patient is anxious or depressed, look for the 'classical' signs of depression, such as early morning waking, diurnal mood variation, loss of interest in previously rewarding activities, etc. If such signs are in evidence, it seems more likely that the patient is depressed than anxious (Carnwath and Miller, 1985).

Intervention and treatment for depression may include the following.

(1) Increase the patient's level of physical activity. Depressed persons typically retreat from physical activity, thus limiting the re-establishment of physical stamina and of motivation to attempt alternative (or even familiar) activities. Clearly some patients will be too weak to undertake much physical exercise, and the emphasis for them will be more appropriately placed on cognitive and social interventions (see below). When patients have the mechanisms of depression explained to them, they can usually understand why the development of physical stamina through increased activity and a gradual programme of physical exercise is an important part of their physical and mental treatment. The principle we attempt to put across to patients is: 'The more you do, the greater the opportunity you have for feeling better.'

(2) Monitor and undermine automatic depressive thoughts. The AIDS epidemic has cast an aura of gloom and despondency around all those associated with

the disease. This has led to people with PGL, ARC and AIDS usually reacting to diagnosis with helplessness and pessimism for the future, seen in patients' 'automatic' assumptions that all efforts to maximise the quality of their (remaining) lives are futile, as they will not help them in the long run. We ask patients to keep a check of all such thoughts, and then proceed to scrutinise and challenge the bases for such defeatist thinking. For example, a terminal cancer patient was recently asked publicly why he kept working on projects he could not hope to finish. He replied that not to do so was rather like coming to a party and not removing his raincoat, not eating, drinking or dancing, because the taxi would be coming to take him home in a few hours, and it would be futile to bother taking part and enjoying himself in the meantime.

(3) Reattribute control in the illness from the virus to the patient. Many patients 'give up' control over their health because of the depressing statistics for outcome after 2 years, and this is frequently associated with a rapid physical decline and appearance of chronic depression. The message that has been emphasised to patients uses the treatment of cancer as a model — i.e. they are told: 'Don't let the virus push you around, you push the virus around.' Imagery techniques, such as the 'Simonton method' (1978) of imagining the virus being crushed and dissolved by the 'life force' in the patient, are encouraged. Similarly, in the treatment of the anxiety accompanying the depression, patients are trained to imagine that the anxiety or despair is a black cloud enshrouding the future. They then visualise blowing the cloud into a small, manageable box set to one side of their imagined landscape of the future, where it rests in a concrete but not so pervasively destructive form. In short, the extent of the anxiety and despair is limited significantly by the patients, allowing them to do other things without these suffocating black clouds hanging over them all the time.

(4) Reintroduce a planned approach to doing things. The withdrawal characteristic of depressed people has been mentioned above. In order to maintain a regimen of increased involvement in routine and pleasurable activities, help patients to list those things they used to do before they were diagnosed or became ill, then devise a plan by which they can gradually work their way up to a realistic amount of future activity. It is important to alternate pleasurable and routine tasks, so that the incentive to persevere is not lost. For example, they might begin by doing the laundry, followed by making an overdue telephone call. Then they might be encouraged to do some shopping, after which they can see a movie or watch television. Taking a walk could be followed by making a small meal, reading a magazine or listening to music, then doing some more shopping, and so on. It is important that new tasks be introduced gradually over a period of days, as health permits. The counsellor should reinforce gains made with praise and encouragement, keeping criticism to a minimum, constructive level. It has been noted by some therapists that patients may encourage overhelping, in which the therapist is asked to do things they could reasonably do for themselves, and this should be discouraged by including such tasks in the planned programme.

(5) Encourage socialisation, perhaps by involving friends and family as 'co-therapists', or by introducing the patient to a relevant support group.

(6) Where possible, encourage the patient to resume employment as soon as realistically possible. The opportunity to re-establish a work regimen provides a good distraction in most cases from the preoccupying worries about AIDS and the future that many patients have to grapple with.

(7) In severe cases of depression, particularly where the patient is becoming obsessional or suicidal, medication may be required. The use of antidepressants, particularly tricyclics, has given good results in many cases, and although the side-effects are fairly easily accommodated, in some cases they may outweigh the benefits otherwise gained. With some antidepressants, administration has been found to induce leucopenia, and so blood tests are necessary with all patients at 4 weeks after initial prescription and at regular intervals thereafter. The other difficulty is the 2-4 week time period required *before* antidepressant effects appear, particularly as graded increases in dosage will usually be necessary to minimise side-effects. In severe cases, where suicide is a possibility, careful patient monitoring is required until effects of medication reliably appear. This may even require emergency psychiatric referral and hospitalisation.

Just as symptom patterns associated with anxiety and depression seem to overlap significantly in this population, so do the components of psychological intervention. All patients respond in idiosyncratic ways, so be prepared to 'chop and change' the nature of the input made as the patient's responses to circumstances change and his individual needs become clear.

Managing Obsessive Disorders

Obsessive disorders, including those with the active compulsive behavioural component, are often seen in the context of depression and anxiety (Carnwath and Miller, 1985). A characteristic of the latter is withdrawal and relative inactivity, and it is frequently the case that the lack of distracting occupations leads to more time spent dwelling on the illness and the bleak prospects for the future. However, such dwelling must be differentiated from those involuntary thoughts and preoccupations with illness and signs of disease that are resisted by the patient without success and that can lead to many hours spent checking for physical signs of deterioration. Where thoughts are involuntary, recurrent, distressing and resisted unsuccessfully by the patient, an obsessive disorder is likely. This phenomenon is increasingly common in these and other patient groups in the context of AIDS (see Chapter 8).

Formulations for the development of obsessive-compulsive disorders vary, but in these states physical checking follows from the involuntary and persistent thought, probably in order to reduce the anxiety about the presence of additional or new infections that the thoughts (or mental images) create. As suggested, the thoughts are resisted by the patient, and so the obsessional thoughts are often described by patients as 'plaguing' them. Not surprisingly, considerable distress follows from this condition, as well as considerable functional disruption, while patients may spend many hours each day looking for confirming evidence on their bodies.

Management of obsessional disorders where compulsive activity is *absent* may include the following.

(1) Reassurance that symptoms described by the patient are not indicative of health decline, where this is the case. Those with PGL will frequently describe faint rashes, pains, visual disturbances, lethargy, etc., which usually follow from chronic, high anxiety, and they must have the symptoms of anxiety explained to them so that future symptoms can be accurately identified by them before they jump to the worst conclusions. Although some individuals are significantly helped by factual explanations and reassurance, with the majority such moves will bring temporary relief only, and other interventions will be required.

(2) Thought stopping, in which the patient is trained to recognise and interrupt the obsessional thoughts when they occur. Thoughts are interrupted by switching immediately to predetermined, potent, pleasantly distracting images, memories, scenes from films, etc., and 'holding on' to the thoughts for a couple of minutes. With practice, thought stopping can provide reliable benefit from intrusive thinking, and produce a lowering of anxiety associated with the possibility of unwanted thoughts recurring.

(3) Avoidance of exposure to media coverage of AIDS. Patients who have managed to achieve reasonable emotional stability after intervention, as well as those suffering obsessional difficulties, will frequently report that the latest news item or newspaper headline undermines their confidence and results in repeated episodes of acute discomfort and worry. Although avoidance is not a conventional suggestion in psychological treatment, the stress generated by often hysterical, misinformed and gloomy media coverage clearly is antitherapeutic, and reducing exposure to this will often result in symptoms of distress being reduced.

(4) In chronic cases where reassurance and other measures bring at best only momentary relief, medication with antidepressants may be the only alternative (especially where the disorder arises in the context of depression). Particular antidepressants, such as clomipramine hydrochloride, have been used with some success in depressed, obsessional patients.

In cases where obsessive thoughts *are* accompanied by compulsive behaviours, most commonly a searching for bodily evidence of infection or cancer, interventions described above may be applied along with *response prevention*. As the term implies, the method involves getting the patient to limit the amount of time given over to bodily checking, so disruption is minimised. The patient may be told to stop checking altogether; or to spend only two minutes checking daily when in the bath; etc. This method has shown considerable benefits in general psychological patient populations (Carnwath and Miller, 1985) and in the context of AIDS.

The management of obsessive disorders and obsessive-compulsive disorders is often very difficult, and reassurance (especially for ARC and PGL patients) and other interventions may often bring only temporary relief. In chronic cases anti-depressant medication may be the only effective solution.

Managing Suicidal Patients

As the numbers of those affected by AIDS, ARC, PGL and HTLV-III infection multiply, the incidence of cases involving suicidal risk also increases. Many of the patients seen fall into well-known suicide risk groups — they are facing recent traumas (diagnosis), many are very depressed, they may have endured the loss of a loved one, they may be living alone and socially isolated, they may have declining physical health and they may be suffering recently imposed financial hardships. At St Mary's Hospital a significant number of those recently diagnosed with AIDS have mentioned to counsellors that they plan to take their own life when and if the pain or discomfort of their condition makes life intolerable, and many have been leading very fast and exciting lives to that point, making their judgement thresholds relatively high. For some who have attempted suicide, the act appears to have been impulsive, without more than a few minutes' prior thought.

When a patient mentions suicide, it is vital to *take him seriously* and not to brush his comments aside. Many will be testing the counsellor in order to see whether they are being taken seriously, and where they feel they are not, fatal consequences may occur. Because attempted suicide is becoming more common-place in this population, intentions for self-harm are routinely (but sensitively) requested. Because the issue creates considerable moral and ethical dilemmas for the therapist, the following response is made: Patients are told that their desire to determine their own death is their right, as long as others are not implicated. Further, where the therapist judges that the likelihood of an attempt is raised in the context of depression or other psychological disorders, the patient is told that all reasonable measures will be taken to prevent it occurring.

This point then raises the issue of management. Where doubt exists over the intentions of the person at risk, emergency psychiatric referral is definitely indicated. Where appropriate, hospitalisation (perhaps with relevant medication) should follow. It is vital for each hospital to have formulated a clear policy on suicidal AIDS-related admissions, and for nursing and other staff to be aware of this. An AIDS isolation ward may not be as appropriate for these purposes as a psychiatric ward.

CONCLUSION

It is clear that the psychological aspects of AIDS, ARC and PGL diagnosis are far-reaching and deeply felt by the patient. It also follows from the discussion above that the consequences of diagnosis provide responsibilities for supervising staff from a wide variety of disciplines within the health care structure, and that staff liaison and co-ordination is a necessity if the consequences are to be kept to a minimum, manageable level. In order to allow this, hospital policies regarding admission and follow-up need to be clearly defined in advance, and necessary training provided as soon as possible to ensure quality control and role definition in counselling and support of the patient. It is unfortunately clear from our experience that too many and too few therapeutic cooks can spoil the patients' broth, yet with a minimum amount of planning and encouragement such an outcome can easily be avoided and the quality of patient life significantly enhanced, even when they may have only a short time left to live. In more fortunate cases strategic input from counsellors and health educators can possibly help to save lives.

REFERENCES

Carnwath, T. and Miller, J. D. (1985). *Behavioural Psychotherapy in Primary Care*. London, Academic Press (in press)

Coates, T. J., Temoshok, L. and Mandel, J. (1984). Psychosocial research is essential to understanding and treating AIDS. *Am. Psychol.*, **39** (11), 1309

Dilley, J. W., Ochitill, H. N., Perl, M. and Volberding, P. A. (1985). Findings in psychiatric consultations with patients with acquired immune deficiency syndrome. *Am. J. Psychiat.*, **142** (1), 82

Green, J. and Miller, J. D. (1985). Male homosexuality and sexual problems. *Br. J. Hosp. Med.*, **33** (6), 353

Miller, J. D. and Green, J. (1985). Psychological support and counselling in acquired immune deficiency syndrome (AIDS). *Genitourin. Med.*, **61**, 273

Miller, D., Green, J., Farmer, R. and Carroll, G. (1985). A 'pseudo-AIDS' syndrome following from a fear of AIDS. *Br. J. Psychiat.*, **146**, 550

Morin, S. F., Charles, K. A. and Malyon, A. K. (1984). The psychological impact of AIDS. *Am. Psychol.*, **39** (11), 1288

Simonton, O. C., Matthews-Simonton, S. and Creighton, J. C. (1978). *Getting Well Again*. Toronto, Bantam Books

Snider, W. D., Simpson, D. M. and Neilsen, S. (1983). Neurological complications of acquired auto immune deficiency syndrome: Analysis of 50 patients. *Ann. Neurol.*, **14**, 403

Wolcott, D. L. (1984). Personal communication

8
Counselling HTLV-III Sero-positives

John Green

INTRODUCTION

It is far from clear exactly how many HTLV-III sero-positive subjects there are in the community. However, it is fairly safe to say that they outnumber those with AIDS by a considerable margin; perhaps 10:1 or even 100:1.

Until recently it has been impractical to routinely screen people for HTLV-III status. With the coming of batch screening methods, this situation will change rapidly. It will soon be possible to screen not only all high-risk subjects coming through a genito-urinary medicine clinic (GUM), but also all blood passing through the Blood Transfusion Service. In the case of GUM patients, there is the issue of whether patients should be routinely screened and, if they are screened, whether they should be told of their status. In the case of Blood Transfusion Service patients, there is the issue of, whether donors should be told of their status, since testing is unavoidable.

Some gay organisations, particularly in the USA, have suggested that subjects should not seek to establish their HTLV-III status, both because there is nothing that can be done to alter that status and because, they argue, the tests available have considerable rates of false-positives and false-negatives. The significance of the test is also in doubt. A positive result probably means that the subject has contacted the virus, but it is usually not clear whether the individual will go on to develop AIDS, and it is not even clear whether the individual is infectious to others. The organisations also point out that subjects who become aware of their HTLV-III status are often very upset and suffer profound psychosocial difficulties.

These arguments are not to be set aside lightly, but there are other considerations which would lead to the opposite conclusion. First, AIDS is a transmissible disease. If it is to be contained, it is important that those who have been infected with the virus should not pass it on to others. Some sero-positive subjects, even those without major symptoms, are clearly infectious to other people, possibly all. Second, there is good reason to believe that, while no currently available treatment can change the HTLV-III status of the infected subject, the subject who has not developed AIDS may be able to reduce the risk of getting the full syndrome by making appropriate changes in life-style. In particular, the acquisition of intercurrent sexually transmitted diseases may worsen immune status, since many of these diseases in themselves affect immune system functioning. It is suspected that they may play a part in the development of full AIDS in those infected with HTLV-III.

Many workers in the field argue that there is little point in testing for HTLV-III status, since, for those in high-risk groups, exactly the same advice prevents acquisition as prevents spread. Consequently, all those in high-risk groups should be counselled in the same way. This argument carries a good deal of weight. However, experience shows that most patients do wish to know their HTLV-III status, and risk-reduction advice carries more weight with persons who are aware that they are sero-positive for HTLV-III. Paradoxically, it is also the author's impression that those who are aware that they are sero-negative are also readier to change their risk behaviours. They feel that they have a lot to lose from not acting to reduce risk.

The psychosocial disturbance which accompanies awareness of being sero-positive cannot be underestimated. For the infected subject, it may mean a radical change in sexual behaviour and also changes in social life, and even in attitudes to self. Counselling can often help to overcome problems arising from such changes. If these problems cannot be overcome, subjects are likely to find it extremely difficult to make the necessary changes. If subjects are to be tested and told their HTLV-III status, it is essential that they should also be offered appropriate advice and counselling.

Not all patients will wish to know their HTLV-III status: clearly the patient ultimately has the right to refuse to know the result of the test, and this right must be respected. It is important to counsel them with respect to safe sex and risk reduction in general. Such patients often have a very shrewd suspicion that they are sero-positive and there is usually no problem in providing risk-reduction information. Additionally, patients who refuse to know are often (though by no means always) anxious and sometimes depressed, and it is important to watch out for this. Fortunately it is rare for patients not to want to know their status.

PRE-COUNSELLING

Because of the above considerations, it is important to see patients before they are tested.

The implications of the test, especially in terms of insurance, financial and employment issues, should be stressed. As much of the information below as possible should be got across. Regardless of whether the result is positive or negative, this advice is important. Vitally, the decision to be tested must be an informed decision.

FACTS AND ISSUES TO GET ACROSS

In counselling sero-positives there are certain facts which it is important to get across.

Facts about the Virus

- The virus is mostly transmitted sexually, but can be transmitted by blood and blood products and by drug abusers sharing needles.

- Being infected with the virus is *not* the same as having AIDS — no one can assure them that they will not get AIDS, but relatively few people infected with the virus do get AIDS.

- There are steps they can take to reduce their risk of getting AIDS, even though they are infected (e.g. safe sex guidelines).

- Even though they do not have AIDS, they may be infectious to others and *those persons* may get AIDS.

It is not usually too difficult to explain the transmission of the virus. The details of transmission are covered in more detail in Chapter 10.

The most difficult point to get across is usually the issue of being infected with the virus but not having AIDS. Most laymen see a one-to-one relationship between infection with an organism and disease. They find it very difficult to separate the two things, while to the counsellor the point appears self-evident. It is tempting to use an analogy to explain the situation but this must be done with caution.

One possible analogy to use is that a person is a 'carrier' for the virus much in the way that someone can be a carrier for hepatitis B. This is an unsuitable analogy for two reasons. First, hepatitis B carriers do not have the symptoms of hepatitis B, although they may have subsequent liver and other problems. The HTLV-III patient, on the other hand, is someone who has been infected with the virus and may subsequently get AIDS — that is, the disease may be active but just not yet have reached the stage of the patient's being symptomatic. Second, the idea of being a 'carrier' is a very emotive one: it makes people think of typhoid carriers. It bears the implication that one is a walking health risk who is inflicting on others something that one has escaped oneself.

A better analogy would probably be with herpes simplex I, in which the subject is infected, may be infectious from time to time and may sometimes be symptomatic. However, this raises a further problem. By bringing in a second disease, patients often become extremely confused. At the end of the day, patients are sometimes confused as to whether they have the disease being discussed in addition to HTLV-III! Particularly with highly anxious patients, complex explanations are probably best avoided.

A further problem arises from the frequent request of patients for information about the probability of their going on to develop AIDS. Various estimates of the rate of AIDS in HTLV-III sero-positives have been proposed varying from 10% to 1%. Because of the long and uncertain incubation period, the relative recency of the disease and the possibility that the latent infection might be triggered by subsequent exposure or illness, it is impossible to give a definitive answer to patients. Nonetheless it is possible to reassure patients that the chances are very good that they will *not* get AIDS. It is also important to stress that they may well be able to reduce their own risk of getting AIDS by making appropriate changes in life-style. This is often a particularly important motivator for changes in sexual behaviour.

Explaining the issue of being able to give someone else AIDS without having it oneself presents similar problems to explaining that of being infected without having the disease. However, it is a far from obvious point to many patients, and needs strong emphasis.

Reduction of Risk

Perhaps the most important issues to get across to sero-positives are those of how they can reduce the risk of transmission of the virus to others, and how they can reduce their own risk of intercurrent sexually transmitted diseases. The other issue which is vital is to reassure the patient of those things which are not a risk. The details of advice on reduction of risk are contained in Chapter 10. However, these are summarised below for convenience.

Sexual

- They should reduce the number of their partners — to one partner if possible.

- They should avoid anal sex altogether.

- If they really cannot manage to avoid anal sex, they should use a condom and extra lubrication. However, they must be advised that this is a risky option.

- They should not transfer body fluids. This includes avoiding 'deep kissing', because saliva may be exchanged.

- They should discuss safe sex guidelines with their existing partner and with prospective partners.

- They should have regular venereological screening.

- They should keep to body rubbing and mutual masturbation.

In covering the sexual guidelines, it is vital to stress the things that they can do as well as the things that they should not do.

Blood

- They must be told that they should not give blood.

- They should not carry an organ donor card.

- They must inform their doctor, particularly where invasive procedures are being undertaken, and their dentist. This information will also help if they subsequently develop health problems.

- They must not have acupuncture, or share razors or toothbrushes or anything likely to be contaminated with blood.

- They should not be shaved in the barber's.

- They need to know about what to do should there be blood spillage (wash surfaces with household bleach, 1 part to 10 parts of water).

- They should not share hypodermic syringes if they are drug abusers.

These issues are covered in more detail in Chapter 10.

What Not to Worry about

- There is no risk from casual contact, shaking hands, kissing on the cheek, just being with people.

- The WC, washbasin and bath present no risk to others.

- The virus is not airborne.

- The virus cannot be caught from cups, cutlery or crockery: no special precautions are required.

- There is no hazard in eating in restaurants, drinking in bars and leading a normal life.

- It is not possible to reinfect oneself (i.e. masturbation is not dangerous).

What to Look out for

It is important to get patients to seek prompt attention for:

- Persistent infections which do not seem to go away.

- Chest infections, particularly with dry cough (i.e. not colds).

- Unexplained skin lesions which persist (not ordinary spots, not cuts or abrasions).

- Unexplained weight loss.

- Persistent or repeated fever.

- Persistent diarrhoea.

- Persistent night sweats.

Presenting such information is difficult. Patients must not be frightened and induced to search repeatedly for minor illnesses and skin blemishes. Muscular aches and pains are a particular problem, since they appear both in patients with persistent generalised lymphadenopathy (PGL) (Metroka *et al.*, 1983) and in patients who are highly anxious. Similarly, fatigue and general malaise appear in patients with PGL and AIDS-related complex (ARC) (covered in more detail below), but also in those who are depressed. Since anxiety and depression are common responses to being sero-positive, there is a real difficulty here.

On the other hand, some asymptomatic sero-positives do subsequently become symptomatic, and of those who are symptomatic some get worse. It is important that they should seek help when this happens, both so that their condition can be monitored and so that early treatment of any physical problems can be started.

GETTING INFORMATION

Additionally there is information which it is helpful for the counsellor to obtain. This serves three purposes: (1) it gives patients the opportunity to voice fears and anxieties they may have; (2) it relates the information provided to the realities of the patient's life and, hence, encourages him to think through likely difficulties; (3) it allows the counsellor to locate likely difficulties and so to help and advise the patient.

The list of questions below is only for guidance; further questioning will depend on the answers to some of these questions. The list of questions is also mainly aimed at homosexual men, since homosexual men form the largest risk group, and the counsellor will need to be selective when dealing with patients from other groups.

Are they homosexual, or heterosexual, or do they engage in both types of sexual behaviour?
Are they intravenous drug users?
Are they haemophilic?

If none of the above, question further to establish likely infection source.

Do they have a stable sexual partner?
If they have a stable sexual partner, are both they and their partner faithful?
How many partners have they had over the past year (male and female)?
How many partners do they usually have per year?
What sexual activities do they engage in?: vaginal intercourse? anal intercourse? oral sex? oral–anal sex? mutual masturbation? body rubbing? insertion of hand into anus ('fisting')? insertion of objects into the anus?
If they engage in anal intercourse, do they use a lubricant, other than saliva?
If they have both homosexual and heterosexual sex, what proportion of sexual activity falls into each category?
In the case of intravenous drug users, do they ever share needles?
Social life: Do they have a network of friends? Do they have non-gay friends?
To what extent do they rely on sex as a source of their social life?
Living: Do they live alone? with friends? with a partner? with family?

Who knows?: Are they openly gay? Do their family know? Do their friends know? Do colleagues at work know? Does their employer know? Does almost no one know?

How do they feel about the news?

What changes will they make in their life-style as a result of the news?

What problems will they have in making these changes?

Are there people they will have to tell — for instance, partners? and how are they likely to take the news?

Additionally, patients need to be assessed for anxiety, depression and obsessional problems; these are covered below.

The questions are aimed at covering several main areas, which risk group they fall into, high-risk behaviours they engage in which may need modification, the availability of non-professional support from friends and relatives, and the patient's reaction to being sero-positive and the practical and emotional difficulties which this will present to him.

In questioning patients it is, of course, important to recognise the fact that sexual activity fulfils many needs other than the need for orgasm. In both homosexuals and heterosexuals it is a source of intimacy, of comfort, of closeness, as well as a way of expressing affection. For many people it is also a primary way of making social contact with others; and if it is removed or curtailed, they may find it difficult to make social contact in other ways.

Apart from the lovers, if they are sympathetic, patients should be urged not to tell others until they have had time to think through and discuss the possible implications.

HELPING THE PATIENT WITH PROBLEMS

Many patients will find that the discussion of the facts about the virus combined with an opportunity to air their problems will be sufficient. However, some patients have specific difficulties either in coming to terms with the diagnosis or with putting into practice the changes in life-style which being sero-positive necessitate.

One of the major difficulties in offering advice to patients is deciding what advice to offer. A key to taking this decision is to break down the patient's problems in a way which makes it clear what issues need to be addressed and the order in which they need to be dealt with. This issue is covered in more detail in Chapter 10, but the application of the method is illustrated in Table 8.1 for a sero-positive patient.

The first step in helping patients is to make a simple list of all the problems which they come up with.

- The problems should be expressed in concrete terms: 'social difficulties' may be accurate but it is uninformative and suggests no solutions, whereas 'meets all partners in gay bars' conveys more information and suggests what line to take in looking for solutions.

- It is important simply to list the problems first and to try to sort them out later.

- It is useful to construct the list with the patient. It helps them to put some structure on their problems, it ensures that the list of problems is correct and the conversation often generates new information.

Once the list of problems has been completed, the next step is to try to find links between problems and to look for possible hypotheses to explain them. In Table 8.1 sleeplessness, lack of appetite and depressed mood seem to go together, and it is reasonable to hypothesise that these are symptoms of a depressed state.

Once each problem has been considered in turn and hypotheses worked out, these can be discussed with the patient. In this case it was very helpful to explain to the patient that sleeplessness and lack of appetite are common in depressed people. It helped to turn something inexplicable into something which the patient could understand.

The next step is to list the assets which the patient has, and the difficulties

Table 8.1 Problem chart for man with PGL

Problems	Links/hypotheses	Possible solutions	Difficulties	Assets
(1) Meets all partners in gay bars – difficult to arrange safe sex	Has not developed other ways of meeting people	Develop alternative social outlets squash club people at work	Only source of social life; known to many people in bars, who expect sex	Assertive; socially skilled; outgoing; likes squash
(2) Wakes early	Depression linked to (3), (4)	Antidepressants; counselling	Dislikes medication	Will take medication if encouraged; puts advice into practice
(3) Feels depressed	Depression linked to (2), (4)	Antidepressants; counselling	As above	As above
(4) Lack of appetite	Depression linked to (2), (3); direct effect of illness	Antidepressants; counselling; encourage to eat appetising diet	Does not feel worth the effort of cooking	Past interest in cookery
(5) Few friends; meets most friends through sex	Linked to (1)	As (1)	As (1)	As (1)
(6) Would like to tell parents he is gay	Not sure how to approach them; not sure of reaction	Get sister to help; role-play how to approach parents with patient	Father frequently comments adversely on homosexuals	Sister knows, and could act as mediator

which he has must be overcome before the problem can be solved. This is most easily seen from Table 8.1.

Once assets and difficulties have been listed, the next stage is to generate possible solutions. It is sensible to generate as many solutions as possible at this stage and to eliminate unsuitable ones later. The patient should be encouraged to try to generate his own solutions because: (a) they are more likely to be suited to his situations, since he knows more about his own life than the counsellor does; (b) he is more likely to follow through things he has suggested himself. However, usually it is necessary for the counsellor to make some input into generating solutions. The counsellor is likely to have seen others with similar problems and has the benefit of knowing how they have handled similar situations.

The final step is to go through the possible solutions and to consider, in the light of assets and difficulties, which solutions are the best, which ones the patient can handle entirely on his own, and which ones the counsellor needs to offer some help on. The issue of treatment is covered in more detail in Chapter 7, but some simple examples of ways in which the counsellor might help include:

- Teaching relaxation to an anxious patient, either directly or by giving him a relaxation tape.

- Role playing with a patient how he is going to tell his parents he is gay, to let the patient have some practice.

- Prescribing antidepressant medication or arranging an appropriate consultation.

- Offering advice on how to make social contacts.

- Encouraging the patient to increase his level of activity if he is depressed, to go out and do things which he has in the past enjoyed or which he has wanted to do in the past but does not feel in the mood to do at the moment.

If a good problem analysis is carried out, the necessary steps are often easy to see. A good analysis also shows the counsellor when referral to someone else is required for specialist help.

Additional Advice

For those who are infected with HTLV-III one of the major difficulties is that they feel that they have no control over their situation. They feel that there is nothing that they themselves can do to reduce their risk of going on to get AIDS. Clearly, one step which they can take is to avoid intercurrent sexually transmitted diseases. However, it is also helpful to suggest other steps which may help to maintain or improve their general health, which will increase their feeling of control and which, at the very least, will cause no harm. Three areas worth covering are diet, exercise and stress.

It is often helpful to get patients to review what they eat and to get them to reduce their intake of processed food and to eat a well-balanced diet with plenty of fresh foods, vegetables and fruit. It is important to establish that there is no special diet which will be helpful, simply a well-balanced diet which they find attractive and enjoyable to eat. Particularly where there are appetite problems, this can prove very helpful.

Moderate exercise, matched to the patient's physical capacity and interests, is also worth while. Swimming or a daily walk is acceptable to most patients and often very enjoyable.

The reduction of stress is also worth achieving. Most people, if they review their work and private lives, can make some reduction in their stressfulness. It is worth going through these areas with patients, making a few simple suggestions and getting them to generate their own ideas. Scheduling time for relaxation is also often helpful, whether this means giving them a relaxation tape to use or finding out how they relax and getting them to schedule specific relaxation time into their day. Half an hour a day simply lying down and listening to music or reading a book can have quite an effect in reducing stress.

These steps should improve general health and subjective well-being and they are something specific which the patients can do to help themselves and so provide some measure of subjective control over events. There is no research evidence that any of these steps actually reduces the chances of going on to get AIDS, but it would not be unreasonable to think that they might, and, at the very least, they would do no one any harm.

PRACTICALITIES

Breaking the News

First Session

There is no easy way to break the news. Ideally the basic information should be got across in the first session. In many busy GUM clinics this may not be possible for reasons of time. However, the basics must be got across, including mode of transmission, the facts that they do *not* have AIDS and that they will probably not get it, and the risks which they present to others and which others present to them.

Many patients are shocked by the news and find it difficult to take in the information. Anxiety blocks the intake of complex information. Therefore it is essential to get patients back in 7–14 days for a longer appointment because:

- It probably won't have been possible to get through the whole of the information at the first session.

- They will probably have some questions.

- They will have had time to think the problem through and will have come up with some problems in changing their behaviour which need to be addressed.

- It is easier to assess any adverse effects in terms of psychological disturbance.

- They will be less anxious and therefore better able to take in the information.

Second Session

It is helpful to go over not only anything which was missed out the first time round, but also, briefly, what was discussed at the first session. Patients who are anxious not only miss a lot of information, but also get it mixed up, and it is essential to be sure that they understand the situation.

If they have told others or tried to change their life-style, it is important to ask them how they got on and what problems they have had. It is important to offer them the opportunity to ask questions and to express their own feelings.

It is important to make it clear that they can come back if they become anxious or depressed, have worries or have physical health problems. Ideally patients should be given a telephone number so that they can ring in. It is often possible to answer questions briefly, to reassure patients or to get them to consult their GPs over the telephone, thus saving the patient worry and the clinic time.

Follow-up

Specific follow-up depends on the exact arrangements of the clinic. Ideally patients should be followed up at 3 months and then at 6-monthly intervals. Naturally this depends on resources. If patients have a good relationship with clinic staff and are well-informed as to what to look out for, they will come in if they run into problems anyway. Even so, it is well worth fixing regular repeat appointments, given the possibility of health problems and the fact that the patients are still infectious.

Some patients will not want to come back. They can best be persuaded to do so by stressing the advantages for them in doing so.

- They can be offered more advice on how to reduce their chances of getting ill.

- Their questions can be answered (ask them to write down any questions which they think of during the period between appointments).

- They will have the opportunity to talk over any outstanding problems. The counsellor has seen others with the same problems and can offer advice based on experience.

- The clinic would like to keep in touch so that if they do have any problems, they can be sure of prompt help.

Depression

Everyone becomes depressed from time to time. However, clinical depression is different in extent and duration from everyday depression. There are several symptoms of depression which it is helpful to look for. These can be conveniently divided into three types – somatic symptoms, cognitive symptoms and behavioural changes.

Somatic Symptoms

One of the commonest symptoms in depression is sleep disturbance – in particular, 'early morning waking'. The patient goes to bed at the normal time but wakes much earlier than normal, at perhaps 4 or 5 a.m., and then cannot go back to sleep. What is being looked for is a recent spontaneous change in sleep patterns. Some people naturally wake very early.

Occasionally, depressed patients sleep far longer than usual when they are depressed, perhaps as much as 30% more, although this pattern is less usual.

Also very common in depression is anorexia, lack of appetite. In severe cases there may be a fair amount of weight loss.

Changes in gastro-intestinal functioning are also often seen – in particular, constipation, but also diarrhoea where the patient is very anxious.

Loss of sexual desire is common in depression, usually without any change in the ability to function sexually when sex takes place.

Some depressed patients develop multiple symptoms which do not seem to fit any disease pattern. It is important here to find out whether the patient has always had multiple health worries and the diagnosis has simply exacerbated these or whether this is a new feature.

One of the problems with identifying somatic symptoms in sero-positives is that the virus itself can cause many of the symptoms which are seen in depression. It can be difficult to decide whether, for instance, the anorexia seen in a patient is the result of infection or of depression. Similarly, gastro-intestinal symptoms are particularly common in homosexual men and it can be difficult to decide what exactly is the cause of these. However, it is the overall pattern which is important in diagnosing depression: the more symptoms the patient has the more likely is the diagnosis.

Cognitive Features

The most obvious symptom of depression is when the patient says that he is depressed, when asked. However, it is possible to be depressed without really being aware of it. The patient may see his position as hopeless and the future as bleak and feel that this is a realistic appraisal of the situation rather than see it as a result of a change in his own thought patterns.

Many depressed patients show obsessional thoughts; these are covered in more detail below.

Pessimism is a key feature of depression: there seems no way out of life's difficulties. The patient may feel excessive guilt about real or imagined past misdemeanours. He may blame himself for all sorts of things — some realistic, some not. With the pessimism and the guilt may come a marked drop in self-esteem: the patient feels worthless and, in extreme cases, a burden to himself and others.

Other changes which patients may complain of are lack of concentration and a slowness of thought. They may also report that they are far more irritable than previously and that they have a feeling of inability to cope with even the smallest tasks.

Crying spells are particularly common in depressed patients, often coming on without warning.

Of great importance in depression is suicide, which gives the condition a sizable mortality rate. Patients who are suspected of being depressed should always be asked whether they feel suicidal and, if so, whether they have actually made any plans to carry out the suicide. Contrary to popular mythology, it is extremely common for suicidal patients to tell others that they are going to kill themselves before doing so. If a patient is planning suicide, an emergency psychiatric consultation is called for.

Finally, a key feature in patients who are depressed is that they cease to enjoy anything. Activities which they previously found pleasurable become a chore, and they may be unable to raise the energy to do any of the things they used to like doing. It is always worth asking patients what they have done over the last 2 weeks which they have actually derived pleasure from. A patient who has enjoyed nothing is very likely to be depressed.

Behavioural Signs

With depression come changes in behaviour, often quite marked. Again, as with somatic symptoms, it is the change in behaviour which is important. Frequently, depressed patients stop doing things, perhaps reducing their activities to the bare minimum. They tend to put things off until tomorrow. Again it is worth asking whether the patients' life has changed recently, whether they have stopped going out or stopped doing things which they used to like.

In extreme cases patients may show motor retardation — that is, a slowness of movement and speech which can make them appear drugged. This is unlikely to be seen in many patients and is so obvious as to be unmissable.

The symptoms of depression are listed in Table 8.2. In identifying patients as depressed there are several factors which it is important to bear in mind. First, it is the overall pattern of symptoms which is important. The more symptoms there are and the more severe they are the more likely the diagnosis and the more severe the depression. Second, it is not just intensity but also duration which is important. Severe depression is easy to recognise. However, quite mild depressions can be a major problem if they persist. The patient may not feel much worse than the interviewer does on a really bad day, but if that depression

Table 8.2   Symptoms of depression

Somatic symptoms
Insomnia; anorexia; constipation; loss of sex drive; multiple physical complaints

Cognitive symptoms
Depressed mood; crying spells; irritability; pessimism; guilt and low self-esteem; difficulty in concentrating; slowness of thought; lack of pleasure in previously enjoyed activities; obsessional thoughts

Behavioural symptoms
Reduction in activity; anxiety

Suicidal thoughts or plans

---

persists for weeks or months, it can be extremely debilitating. It is worth enquiring of depressed patients how many days over the last 2 weeks they have felt low. If they have felt low every day, then they may well have a problem. Third, suicidal thoughts, especially where the patient is actively planning, should always be taken seriously. Finally, anxiety is particularly common in depressed patients; this subject is covered in more detail in the next section.

Treatment

Depression is treated in two different ways: by psychological means and by the use of drugs. For mild depression with clear precipitating factors, psychological treatments are often helpful used alone. For more severe depression, while psychological approaches are effective, it is often easiest and most comfortable for the patient to use a combination of drugs and counselling.

The tricyclic antidepressants are fairly safe drugs. They are non-addictive and produce good results in a majority of cases. It is important to stress to the patient, when prescribing, that the drugs (a) are not tranquillisers and (b) will not have an immediate effect: the lifting of the depression may take some time to occur, perhaps 2-4 weeks before the patient feels much better. Side-effects, which are usually mild, frequently appear much earlier and, hence, patients must expect an initial period in which they may experience some side-effects without apparently getting benefit.

Anxiety

Anxiety is extremely common. Under many circumstances it is quite normal — for instance, when going into an examination, when called upon to make a speech before a large audience or when told one is HTLV-III sero-positive. In other cases the anxiety is out of proportion to the immediate threat — for instance, in cases of agoraphobia or lift or tube phobia.

Anxiety management techniques are effective in reducing anxiety, not just in cases where the fear is out of proportion but also in cases where it is reasonable (Carnworth and Miller, 1985). The techniques of anxiety management are covered in detail in Chapter 7. These are fairly easily applicable in a brief consultation and often very effective.

Table 8.3 lists the most common symptoms of anxiety. The somatic symptoms are those of the 'fight or flight response' — that is, they prepare the body

Table 8.3 Symptoms of anxiety

Somatic symptoms
Cardiovascular: increased heart rate; 'pounding heart' (probably increased cardiac output); coldness and whiteness of extremities; flushing
Respiratory: breathlessness; tightness in the chest; chest pain; hyperventilation
Muscular: tension headache; aches and pains in the muscles; increased tremor; shaking
Gastro-intestinal: dry mouth; nausea; diarrhoea; poor appetite
Sleep: disturbed sleep (difficulty in getting to sleep, light sleep with frequent waking, vivid dreams); fatigue
Libido: loss of desire; impotence; retarded ejaculation
Other: dizziness; tingling in the extremities; sweating — particularly from the hands and feet but also general

Cognitive symptoms
Subjective fear and anxiety; constant worrying thoughts about the significance of minor symptoms; poor concentration; hypersensitivity to noise and distraction; feelings of being unreal or of the world being unreal

Behavioural symptoms
The anxiety may be focal — i.e. it may be linked to particular situations or circumstances, in which case the patient may show avoidance of the feared situation

for muscular effort. The rise in heart rate increases blood flow; sweating prepares for the dissipation of the heat generated by muscular effort; sweating on the palmar and plantar surfaces improves grip and protects against the skin being torn (hydrated skin is more resistant to tearing); and blood flow to the digestive system is reduced preparatory to increased demand for the musculatory system. There also tends to be a rise in the respiration rate. Where this is extreme, hyperventilatory symptoms may appear, including dizziness, pallor in the extremities, feelings of faintness and, sometimes, tingling or numbness in the hands and feet. Hyperventilation leads to a feeling of tightness in the chest and of breathlessness which tends to make the patient overbreathe even more.

It is worth explaining in detail to the patient the nature of his symptoms, since they are often dramatic and the patient may feel that he is very ill, going mad or even dying if he has panic attacks.

One of the difficulties in diagnosing anxiety in HTLV-III sero-positives is that the virus in itself can cause some of the symptoms which are seen in anxiety (Chapter 1).

Treatments for anxiety are dealt with in detail in Chapter 10.

Obsessions

Obsessions fall into two categories: (1) obsessional behaviour and (2) obsessional thoughts.

In obsessional behaviour the patient feels obliged to repeat some act or behaviour in a very stereotyped way. A good example is the common childhood experience of stepping over cracks in the pavement. Another is the person who sets off on holiday, gets half-way down the road and then goes back to check. He knows that he has switched off the gas really, but feels that he will not be able to relax unless he checks. A common form of obsessional behaviour in sero-positives is checking the body for rashes or blemishes. Checking may take up many minutes or hours, and the patient may become very distressed but still feel that he must go through the checking until he is absolutely sure he has nothing abnormal on his skin. The behaviour often has a strong ritualistic flavour: the patient may feel that he must start with the feet and work up the body in a particular order, for instance.

Obsessional thoughts are stereotyped thoughts which go round and round in the patient's mind. They often have a very unpleasant content — for instance, thoughts of death and dying. Quite often they involve a sort of mental checking. Patients may go over and over their past sex life to try to work out whether any of their past partners showed any signs of ill-health. Or they may try to work out whether they have done anything inadvertently which may have exposed their family or friends to the virus — cutting themselves, for instance. At the extreme, patients may have to go through a sort of mental ritual, feeling they have to start with their very first sexual partner and working through the rest in order. They may even feel that if they make a mistake, they have to go back and start again from the beginning.

Obsessional thoughts and behaviours are often seen in depression and lift with the depression. It is also often very difficult to distinguish obsessions from anxiety. Anxious patients often worry continuously and may check their body frequently. This sort of behaviour often shades into frank obsessionality, and it is difficult to say where one ends and the other begins. However, obsessions may be seen as a quite separate problem in someone who is not depressed and who is not unduly anxious, except in so far as having obsessions tends to lead in itself to anxiety. The treatment of obsessions is covered in detail in Chapter 7.

SPECIAL PROBLEMS

The Symptomatic Patient

The advice given to patients who are HTLV-III sero-positive and also have symptoms is, in general, the same as that given to asymptomatic sero-positives, and the same procedures and considerations apply. The most common symptoms seen are those of persistent generalised lymphadenopathy. In some patients PGL seems to be an end state in itself: the lymph glands remain swollen and the patient gets neither better nor worse. In a few cases the lymphadenopathy appears to resolve. A fairly substantial proportion of patients get worse and go on to develop AIDS. Even so, those moving from PGL to AIDS appear to be in the minority. However, the presence of PGL forces the counsellor to a less optimistic assessment of the likelihood of a patient's developing AIDS.

It is important to explain these facts to patients and to stress that having PGL does not necessarily mean that they will get AIDS. Some patients have PGL and a fairly large number of different physical problems, including persistent infections and skin rashes. At the same time they do not fulfil the CDC criteria for AIDS. This state of affairs is sometimes described as the AIDS-related complex. In some cases the division of these patients from AIDS patients is probably one of definition; in others the difference in nomenclature reflects a real difference in their state of health.

When counselling symptomatic patients, important factors to look out for are:

- Their chances of developing AIDS are greater than those of an asymptomatic patient. Exactly how much greater will vary from patient to patient, and, hence, it is absolutely vital that the counsellor should be well briefed on the clinical state of the patient. Of patients with PGL alone, only a minority will go on to get AIDS, as far as is known at the moment. For a patient with multiple persistent infections and other symptoms, the outlook is not so good.

- The presence of symptoms serves as a constant reminder to the patient that he is infected with the virus.

- It is important to keep the patient fully informed at each point about his clinical state. It is important to be as honest as possible in this respect, even when the news is bad. If patients are to believe the counsellor when the news is good, they must be clear that they will be told the worst when the news is bad. It is often the counsellor, after liaison with the appropriate clinical staff, who will inform patients about the details and the significance for them of tests and diagnoses, so that it is important to have this material available.

- The importance of the patient's keeping in touch with the hospital cannot be overstressed. Only in this way can changes in clinical state be monitored and early treatment of infections undertaken.

- Patients with PGL and ARC may need more frequent meetings with the counsellor than are likely to be needed by the majority of asymptomatics.

- In many cases of symptomatic PGL the same procedures are likely to be required as in dealing with AIDS patients (see Chapter 7).

The 'Worried Well'

In addition to those patients who are infected with the virus, a large number of people in the community are worried that they may have AIDS. These patients turn up from time to time seeking reassurance and help. Handling these patients is discussed in Chapter 9.

Advising Sero-negatives

Many people in high-risk groups wish to reduce their risk of acquiring the virus. Essentially the procedures for this group are much the same as for those who are known to be sero-positive. Clearly, the same procedures prevent someone acquiring the virus and also passing it on to others.

Clear concise information on the virus, on its mode of transmission and on ways of reducing risk need to be given. It is helpful to discuss with patients practical difficulties which they feel they may encounter in trying to keep to safe sex procedures, in the same way as with sero-positives.

The majority of people seeking advice on reducing their risk are simply responsible people who wish to take all possible steps to ensure their safety. With clear advice they are able to make an informed decision as to what changes they wish to make in their life-style. It is, however, worth bearing in mind that a minority of patients coming to seek advice are likely to be highly anxious, although they may present initially as simply seeking advice. It is always worth enquiring whether they worry a lot about AIDS. Clearly, someone who worries most of the time about AIDS is not simply concerned – he has a specific AIDS fear, and the possibility of anxiety, depression or obsessions needs to be looked into (Miller *et al.*, 1985).

REFERENCES

Carnworth, T. and Miller, D. (1985). *Behavioural Psychotherapy in Primary Care.* London, Academic Press (in press)

Metroka, C. E. and Cunningham-Rundles, S. *et al.* (1983). Generalised lymphadenopathy in homosexual men. *Ann. Int. Med.*, **99**, 585

Miller, D., Green, J., Farmer, R. and Carroll, G. (1985). A 'pseudo-AIDS' syndrome following from fear of AIDS. *Br. J. Psychiat.*, **146**, 550

9

The Worried Well

David Miller

INTRODUCTION

Previous chapters have discussed the psychological consequences of having AIDS, ARC, PGL, of being sero-positive for the HTLV-III virus and of being in a high-risk group. However, the AIDS epidemic has become a cause of considerable functional and psychological disruption for those individuals who, for varying reasons, perceive themselves to be at high risk irrespective of their proximity to the high-risk categories. These persons are known as the 'worried well': they are worried about developing AIDS, and they are well in that they show no objective signs of AIDS-related illness.

The worried well present for many reasons — for example, because they may have had sex with a bisexual man or woman in the past, because they are homosexual or have had a history of (periodic) homosexual activity (frequently involving only low-risk activity), or because they are psychologically vulnerable personalities who have responded to the AIDS reports from sections of the media which have been less than well informed or sensitive in their coverage. The clinical presentation of such persons typically includes acute and sometimes chronic anxiety, with panic attacks, agitated depression and obsessional disorders involving a morbid preoccupation with the prospect of developing AIDS, together with hypochondriacal reactions to autonomic anxiety symptoms which are perceived as evidence of frank viral infection and prodromal AIDS.

In this context, patients will often have a distorted view of infection risks and of their own personal vulnerability to transmission of the AIDS virus. This may be largely due to the symptoms associated with their anxieties. Miller *et al.* (1985) have described a 'pseudo-AIDS' syndrome affecting the worried well, in which their fears of infection generate many of the anxiety symptoms that appear to mimic the prodromal features of AIDS, such as sweating, lethargy, rashes, appetite loss and weight loss. The appearance of such symptoms, in turn, appears to 'confirm' their worst fears, thus making the symptoms worse and leading to frank psychological or psychiatric disturbance, together with considerable functional disruptions of the types discussed elsewhere (see Chapter 7) (Morin *et al.*, 1984).

MANAGEMENT OF THE WORRIED WELL

The psychological management of the worried well essentially follows the same format as for sero-positives, PGLs, ARC and frank AIDS patients (see Chapters 7 and 8). The difference in management concerns the uncertainty of the patients' actual contact with the virus. Frequently, patients will accept only the results of HTLV-III antibody screening as confirmation of their viral status, irrespective of the reassurance that may follow from a close analysis of their sexual history excluding risk of virus transmission. In more severe cases the patient may focus on the relative unreliability of the blood screening test, and the obsessional difficulties will reappear after an initial period of reassurance. The authors know of some patients who have gone from clinic to clinic in search of a test result that confirms their worst fears. Others respond to the 'standard' format of intervention, even when suicidal tendencies have resulted from the anxieties over infection (Miller *et al.*, 1985).

Discussion

The first step is to discuss the nature of the patient's anxieties, so that his or her concerns may be ventilated. Many of those within this patient group, such as married women and bisexual men, and others who may have become fearful of their health status following covert sexual activity (e.g. 'closet' homosexuals), will have been unable to discuss their anxieties with partners, spouses, friends or family for fear of being 'discovered', and the opportunity to talk about this will in itself provide considerable relief. For others, such as homosexual men who may have had multiple sexual partners in the past, the opportunity to ventilate is novel, as their friends and acquaintances may have avoided such discussion, or they may have told the patient not to talk about AIDS because they do not wish to be reminded about their own level of risk, or are perhaps too frightened to discuss it.

Assessment of Risk and HTLV-III Exposure

During the ventilation stage, the degree of high-risk sexual activity to which the patient has been exposed can be ascertained. In some cases, perhaps where mutual masturbation only or uncomplicated vaginal intercourse (e.g. with the use of condoms) has taken place, patients can be reassured that they have not been exposed to transmission of the virus. In other cases, perhaps where an opportunistic infection has been acquired, or the 'casual' lover has become ill with AIDS-related symptoms, or where high-risk activity with a member of a high-risk group has taken place within the last 5-10 years, it may be necessary to request a medical examination (see Chapter 1). If the patient asks for blood anti-body screening, or it is indicated by examination, the full significance and possible consequences of a positive result should be made clear to him in advance. A useful format for conversational screening of risk is presented in Chapter 10.

In many cases the patient will already have had such a screening, and the assessment of risk may be necessary simply as a reassuring mechanism in therapy. However, where a patient has been very recently at risk there may not have been time for measurable sero-conversion to have occurred, and this will have to be explained to the patient and a follow-up appointment for screening will have to be made.

Provision of Information

Once the absence of risk and exposure has been determined, it is necessary to provide clear and repeated reassurance that the patient is not HTLV-III sero-positive, together with information about how to avoid the risk of future exposure. Where the patient has become worried because of sexual activity outside an established relationship, clearly the simplest course is to suggest future monogamy (preferably to both partners). Where the worried patient is having sexual relations with an identified HTLV-III-antibody-positive partner (e.g. the wife of a haemophiliac, a homosexual lover), it is desirable to provide information on safer sex procedures and precautions (see Chapter 10).

Where a patient comes from a low-risk group, he or she should be told exactly why he or she cannot have caught the virus, and also told about the nature of the virus in much the same way as is suggested for sero-positives. One patient seen by the authors felt that she was at risk because her next-door neighbour was a homosexual man and she was afraid of having caught the virus by having tea with him. A clear explanation of why this could not have happened cured her fears.

Other writers (Miller and Green, 1984; Morin et al., 1984) have noted that in some cases the worried patient will actually avoid becoming informed about AIDS and procedures for minimising risk because doing so is simply too frightening. In such cases clear discussion will usually help to overcome such resistance, particularly where the news is good!

Assessment for Psychological and Functional Disturbances

As with the difficulties arising for those directly affected by HTLV-III infection, the worried well present with considerable problems of an emotional, psychological, domestic, occupational and social variety (Miller and Green, 1985; Morin et al., 1984). The severity and significance of such difficulties need to be established so that appropriate management can be instituted by the therapist, and appropriate responses can be made by the patient in an effort to resume control and perspective on circumstances. Detailed discussion of the assessment and management methods for anxiety, depression, obsessional disorders and problem-solving procedures is presented in Chapters 7 and 8.

Confirmation of Understanding

During and after the necessary information and therapist intervention, patients should be routinely asked whether they are happy with the explanations and information they have received. Most patients should be quite content with the rational and informed intervention of the counsellor or therapist, but some may be hesitant to voice nagging doubts, and intervention will therefore cease to show any positive effect. This may be simply because the therapist has overlooked some essential discussion points, or it may be because the patient has developed a chronic psychological difficulty, which may then require specialist psychological or psychiatric attention. In such cases the appropriate referral should be made as soon as possible.

It is also worth bearing in mind that for some patients worrying about AIDS is only the last stage in a long line of persistent health worries. For the very hypochondriacal patient, diseases which are prominent in the media can become a focus for general anxieties and obsessions. At the turn of the century the majority of those with hypochondriacal anxieties seem to have felt that they had tuberculosis, and more recent media reports have generated considerable patient obsessions about the personal inevitability of breast cancer. Now many patients fear they may have AIDS.

In these circumstances patients should always be asked whether they worry frequently about their health and how often they consult their GP. Health worries are also quite common in the depressed patient, emphasising the importance of screening for possible depression.

CONCLUSION

Even given the severity of disturbance in some patients, very few of the worried well do not actually respond to simple, clear and patiently given information about the disease, together with firm assertions that they are not infected. When backed up by clear advice on how to avoid the possibility of future exposure to HTLV-III virus, intervention can frequently be terminated after three or four sessions.

REFERENCES

Miller, D. and Green, J. (1984). The AIDS epidemic: Advising homosexual men on reducing their level of risk. *Br. J. Sexual Med.*, **11** (107), 106

Miller, D. and Green, J. (1985). Psychological support and counselling in acquired immune deficiency syndrome (AIDS). *Genitourin. Med.*, **61**, 273

Miller, D., Green, J., Farmer, R. and Carroll, G. (1985). A 'pseudo-AIDS' syndrome following from a fear of AIDS. *Br. J. Psychiat.*, **146**, 550

Morin, S. F., Charles, K. A. and Malyon, A. K. (1984). The psychological impact of AIDS. *Am. Psychol.*, **39** (11), 1288

10

Reduction of Risk in High-risk Groups

John Green

INTRODUCTION

Since there is currently no cure for AIDS or for infection by the HTLV-III virus, prevention is a matter of vital concern. In large part this depends on health education. It is vital that those infected with the virus should not pass it on and that those at high risk of acquiring the virus should be aware of ways in which they can reduce their level of risk. This chapter aims to cover the information which it is necessary for patients to be aware of and provides at least some of the details necessary to answer questions which patients may have.

HTLV-III is a blood-borne virus. It appears that there are three main ways in which the virus is likely to be transmitted in the UK.

(1) *Sexually*   The majority of cases of AIDS originating in the USA and in Europe are in homosexual men. It is clear that the virus can be spread sexually and probable that certain sexual behaviours — anal intercourse, in particular — are particularly important in the spread of the disease. The virus can also be spread by heterosexual vaginal intercourse, although cases occurring in this way are less common at present.

(2) *Through blood transfusions and blood products*   Haemophiliacs in both the UK and the USA show high rates of antibodies to HTLV-III. This is the result of their using contaminated factor VIII or factor IX. The virus can also be spread by blood transfusions with whole blood.

(3) *Other sources of risk*   The other major route of infection is through infected blood entering a person's body. The most obvious example of this type of infection is needle-stick accidents in medical and nursing staff. The rate of sero-conversion is very low in these cases, so that these accidents do not appear to be a major source of HTLV-III infection. Intravenous (i.v.) drug abusers have become infected through the sharing of syringes. Theoretically, other invasive procedures where contamination with infected blood occurs may be a source of infection.

SEXUAL ACTIVITY AND HTLV-III

The group at most risk of acquiring HTLV-III infection are homosexual men: in the USA over 70% of all cases of AIDS are in homosexual or bisexual men; the figure for cases of European origin is 87% (CDC figures). There seem to be several reasons for this.

(a) Surveys of homosexual men have shown that, in general, subjects had had more sexual partners than heterosexual men. Surveys carried out in the USA (e.g. Saghir and Robins, 1973; Bell and Weinberg, 1978) show a pattern of large numbers of sexual partners. In the Saghir and Robins study 94% of homosexual men had had more than 15 partners and 75% more than 30 partners, compared with 21% and 0%, respectively, among heterosexuals. Studies carried out in STD clinics in the UK (Murray-Sykes, 1983; Roberts, 1985) show a similar pattern among UK homosexual men. These studies used highly selected samples of men in the case of the USA samples, drawn from 'scene' gays in areas of the country which might be expected to attract men looking specifically for a free-wheeling life-style. The UK samples referred to are also unlikely to be typical, for obvious reasons. It is not clear to what degree samples reflect the sexual behaviour of homosexual men in general. Experience with the sexual partners of homosexual men seeking treatment for sexual dysfunction at St Mary's Hospital suggests that a proportion of homosexual men have relatively few sexual partners.

Even so, it is clear that a sizable proportion of homosexual men are likely to have far more different partners than the majority of heterosexuals. The risk of acquiring any sexually transmitted disease rises with the number of partners a person has. This is reflected in studies showing high levels of STDs in homosexual men (Judson et al., 1977; Ritchey, 1977; Sohn and Bibilotti, 1977). There is some evidence that homosexual AIDS patients have had more sexual partners than have homosexual controls (Jaffe et al., 1983).

(b) The specific sexual activities of homosexual men may put them at more risk than heterosexuals (Marmor, 1984; Marmor et al., 1984). Jaffe et al. (1983) showed in an early case-control study that insertion of the tongue and hand into the rectum was more common in AIDS cases than in controls and that they had had a higher rate of anal intercourse.

It seems likely that anal intercourse and other sexual activities likely to involve rectal trauma provide particularly favourable conditions for transmission of the virus. Jaffe et al. grouped these behaviours as 'exposure to faeces'. However, it seems likely that the major risk factor is rectal bleeding, which always accompanies anal intercourse even where it is not obvious to the participants. Clearly, insertion of the hand makes rectal trauma almost inevitable.

(c) Another issue is that it seems likely that certain co-factors increase the likelihood of the development of AIDS in those who are infected with HTLV-III. A prime suspect must be intercurrent sexually transmitted diseases. As noted above, some homosexual men have a history of repeated STDs. The existence of co-factors would also explain why only a minority of people infected with the virus go on to develop AIDS.

Safer Homosexual Sex

Risk reduction depends on a change in sexual behaviour aimed at reducing the risk of acquisition of HTLV-III and intercurrent sexually transmitted diseases. The issue of advising homosexual men on making their sexual behaviour safer has been covered to some extent in Chapter 8. This section aims to provide the rationale for the advice given and to provide some information on the sorts of difficulties which have to be overcome if a man is to change his sexual behaviour.

Reduction of Number of Sexual Partners, Preferably to One

Clearly, in a totally monogamous relationship with no other risk factors present there is no risk of acquisition of the virus. The difficulty is that such relationships seem to be rare among those homosexual men who have been studied in detail. Bell and Weinberg (1978) found that only 10% of their sample were in a stable, more or less faithful, relationship. On the other hand, there is evidence that a large proportion of homosexual men have a stable partner at one time or another (Saghir and Robins, 1973; Weinberg and Williams, 1974; Murray-Sykes, 1983). Therefore, it is a step which a large number of homosexual men probably have the potential to take if they wish to.

Where this is not a step which a man wishes to take, there is still an advantage in reducing the number of partners. Some agencies have suggested that it would be worth while for a homosexual man to examine a prospective partner closely before having sex, in order to establish that he is in good health. It is unclear how effective this would be. Not only are many HTLV-III sero-positives asymptomatic, but also they may be unaware that they are sero-positive. Although an inspection of a partner may reveal signs of Kaposi's sarcoma or of active syphilis and other STDs, it is clearly impractical for a man to carry out a full medical on a prospective partner. Wright and Wright (1985) report that gay men in San Francisco are developing a preference for men who are well-built or slightly obese, since weight loss is associated with AIDS. The difficulties this is likely to present to slim healthy men are obvious!

Avoidance of Anal Intercourse, Oral-Anal Contact and Insertion of Objects or Hand into Anus

Available studies show that anal intercourse is almost universal among homosexual men. The majority engage in both active (insertor) and passive (insertee) intercourse. In view of its very high risk, it is important that a homosexual man should give up anal intercourse, as well as insertion of the hand into the rectum ('fisting') and oral-anal contact ('rimming'). The exception is where the homosexual man has a stable faithful monogamous relationship with one other man, in which there is little risk.

For many gay men this is unacceptable. For the subject who really does not wish to give up anal intercourse, condoms may provide some degree of protection. However, there are a number of problems with condoms. The first is that there is no clear evidence that they do, in fact, prevent transmission of HTLV-III. They reduce transmission of other STDs, so by analogy they may reduce the risk of HTLV-III, but this is not proven. Most condoms are designed with vaginal intercourse in mind. They have a significant failure rate, especially when not used exactly as specified by the manufacturer (i.e. if fitted before an erection is fully present or if the subject withdraws the penis during intercourse). The mechanical stresses in anal intercourse are probably greater and there is evidence, from anal intercourse by female prostitutes, at least, that a high failure rate may be expected (Barton, 1985). Some condoms are specifically designed to be tougher, but where these are made from natural membranes, the situation with respect to passage of the virus is even more unclear.

If a homosexual man wishes to use a condom, it should be used with a good lubricant, preferably one of those made specifically for vaginal intercourse. Saliva is the most frequently used lubricant and has particularly poor properties in that role.

However a condom is used, and whatever extra precautions are used, it is clear that the use of a condom is on present knowledge a poor substitute for cutting down on anal intercourse. Other forms of contact with the anus are to be totally avoided: for instance, there is no way in which oral–anal sex can be regarded as anything but a high-risk activity. Nevertheless, where giving up anal sex is not acceptable, the use of a condom should be encouraged.

Avoidance of Oral Sex

HTLV-III can be isolated from, and transmitted by, semen. The risk of transmission by this route during oral sex is difficult to assess. However, it is potentially a risk. Even withdrawing the penis before ejaculation does not totally avoid risk, since many men produce some secretion from the penis prior to ejaculation taking place, sometimes quite a time before.

The HTLV-III virus has been found in the saliva of some sero-positive men. How infectious it is in saliva is not clear, and there are no cases in which infection can be clearly attributed to contact with saliva. At the moment it is not possible to assume that there is no risk of transmission through saliva.

Under the circumstances it is clear that oral sex is to be avoided in either the fellator or the fellatee role.

Avoidance of Transmission of Body Fluids

Since saliva is known to contain HTLV-III virus in some sero-positives, deep (lingual) kissing, in which large amounts of saliva may be exchanged, should be avoided. So should activities in which other body fluids may be exchanged, including semen smearing and coprophagia. Although there is no evidence that the virus is present in urine, it is probably wise to avoid 'water sports' — sexual activities involving urinating onto the partner, particularly into his mouth or rectum. Other viruses (e.g. CMV) may be present in urine.

Discussion of Safe Sex Guidelines with Partners or Prospective Partners

It is clearly important in any sexual relationship that partners should agree on what sexual activities are or are not acceptable. It is likely to be easier for a man to discuss safer sex with an existing partner. It is rather more difficult to discuss safe sex with a prospective partner. Even so, it is a matter of considerable importance that this should occur. Patients report that rehearsing the discussion of safer sex prior to involvement with a prospective partner is extremely helpful in assisting them in dealing with the situation.

Regular Venereological Screenings

The use of regular venerological screenings is important. It means that intercurrent sexually transmitted diseases can be picked up and treated early. It means that a sero-negative man can reassure himself that he remains so or will know if he becomes infected with the virus. It also means in symptomatic sero-positives that there is a much higher probability that any symptoms that may develop, particularly opportunistic infections, can be recognised and treated at an early stage.

Keeping to Mutual Masturbation and Body Rubbing

Where a man is unable to locate a single faithful partner, the risk of contracting the virus, and most other sexually transmitted diseases, can be reduced if he confines his sexual activity to mutual masturbation or reaching orgasm by rubbing the penis against the skin of the partner (as opposed to mucous membrane). Intact skin is a good mechanical barrier against infection with most organisms, although there are exceptions, and has antibacterial and antiviral properties arising from natural flora and various chemical mechanisms. Clearly, where there is actual skin damage on, say, the hands, either through injury or through skin lesions such as eczema, sexual activity involving these areas is to be avoided.

Nonetheless, mutual masturbation and body rubbing, though not preferred sexual behaviours for many homosexual men, are often acceptable forms of sexual activity. For the man who cannot or will not avoid casual contacts, they provide a way of reducing risk of acquisition or transmission considerably.

Heterosexual Intercourse

Although most AIDS patients in the USA and Europe are homosexual men, AIDS is transmissible in vaginal intercourse, both from men to women and almost certainly from women to men. It has been suggested that, like hepatitis B, the virus is less easily transmissible through vaginal than anal intercourse. However, there have been a considerable number of cases of heterosexually transmitted AIDS, and it is to be expected that this number may increase in the future. Reports from the USA suggest that there has been a recent increase in heterosexual cases, particularly in women.

In Central Africa the male:female ratio is approaching 6:4. It is highly likely that the disease is heterosexually transmitted in such cases. The question as to whether the African AIDS virus is a different strain of HTLV-III remains unanswered. There is no reason to suppose that AIDS could not become a major sexually transmitted disease in Europe and the USA.

For a sero-positive subject engaging in heterosexual activity, the same considerations apply to oral sex, anal intercourse and other sexual activities as apply to someone engaging in homosexual activity, with the addition that it is probably wise to avoid vaginal intercourse. This is an important issue, and it is necessary to be aware that a considerable proportion of homosexual men enagage in heterosexual intercourse from time to time (Green and Miller, 1985), so that they need to be aware that a considerable proportion of homosexual men engage in heterohigh-risk groups. For the man or woman who is unable or unwilling to give up vaginal intercourse, the use of condoms may possibly reduce risk and their rate of breakage may be lower. However, the protective value of condoms is unproven in preventing HTLV-III transmission.

Where either the woman or her partner are sero-positive, prevention of pregnancy must be a primary consideration. There is every reason to believe that the fetus can be infected with HTLV-III (see Chapter 3). There have now been a considerable number of paediatric cases of AIDS (CDC statistics). Where pregnancy does occur, the possibility of termination may have to be considered carefully with the couple. It follows that even where a condom is being used, it would be wise for couples to combine it with another method of contraception to provide extra protection.

TRANSMISSION THROUGH BLOOD OR BLOOD PRODUCTS

The risk of getting AIDS through a single UK blood transfusion is extremely low and with the introduction of screening is probably not worth worrying about. Clearly, transfusions are not given except where really necessary, and the risks from not having the transfusion are likely to outweigh many times over any slight risk of being infected with HTLV-III. There have been cases of transfusion-linked HTLV-III infection both in the UK and in the USA, but it is hoped that these will become much rarer in the future.

Unfortunately the risks of transmission of HTLV-III to haemophiliacs receiving either factor VIII or factor IX are much greater. The pooling of blood to obtain clotting agents significantly increases the risk that any individual using those agents will be infected. In 1984 34% of a sample of 184 UK haemophiliacs receiving pooled clotting factor were sero-positive (Cheingsong-Popov *et al.*, 1984).

Until recently much of the clotting factors used in the UK has been imported from the USA. A proportion of this was infected with HTLV-III. Shortly the UK should become self-sufficient in blood products. This, combined with screening of UK blood, should significantly reduce the risk to haemophiliacs. There is also evidence that the use of heat-treated blood products may reduce the risk of infection by the virus.

Despite high rates of sero-conversion among haemophiliacs, the risks from HTLV-III are far outweighed by those from the effects of haemophilia itself. Haemophiliacs should *not* change their treatment regimen without careful consultation with their medical advisors. Clear advice has been offered in a booklet designed for haemophiliacs (Jones, 1985).

The issue of sexual activity for haemophiliacs is a particularly difficult one. Many are married or have stable sexual partners, but are unable to change their major risk factor — the use of blood products. The only safe step is for them to adopt the guidelines on sex outlined above. Many haemophiliacs do not wish to completely eliminate vaginal intercourse and, once the haemophiliac and partner are fully informed of the risk, they may choose, as do many others, to use condoms. The importance of avoiding pregnancy must be stressed, and this frequently causes great distress.

OTHER SOURCES OF RISK

The other major way in which HTLV-III can be transmitted is by infected blood reaching the blood of the recipient. The routes by which this can occur can be summarised as follows.

Intravenous Drug Abuse

Intravenous drug abusers form about 17% of USA AIDS cases. The majority of these cases cluster in New York. Currently i.v. drug abusers represent less than 1% of cases originating in Europe. Cheingsong-Popov *et al.* (1984) reported that only 1.5% of 269 UK drug abusers showed HTLV-III antibodies. On the other hand, this is a group in which an increase in sero-positivity is to be expected in the future.

The major factor in spread in i.v. drug abusers would seem to be needle sharing, as in hepatitis B. It is possible that one reason for the clustering of cases in New York is the existence of 'shooting galleries', where needles and syringes may be hired and are frequently shared by large numbers of users. Available evidence suggests that UK i.v. drug abusers also share needles frequently (Mulleady and Green, in preparation), although there is nothing in the UK to compare with the 'shooting galleries'. Most sharing is done with one other person, although some users do take drugs in a group. 'Pumping', moving blood in and out of the syringe, clearly increases risk of transmission. Obviously, if needle and syringe sharing were eliminated, the risk of HTLV-III transmission in i.v. drug abusers would be substantially reduced. Unfortunately, few i.v. drug abusers seem particularly concerned about health risks, as has been shown in the case of hepatitis B, which remains a major risk in drug users. Nonetheless, it is vital that those dealing with drugs should endeavour to persuade their patients to reduce needle sharing.

A sizable proportion of i.v. drug users, particularly women but sometimes men, earn the money for drugs from prostitution. They therefore represent a potentially important route for the transmission of HTLV-III to others. It is difficult to be optimistic about the chances of implementing 'safe sex' guidelines in this situation. Nonetheless, it is important to try.

Opiate use reduces sex drive, and so many drug users have relatively little sexual activity. Where the user ceases to use drugs, however, the drive is likely to return. Therefore it is important to monitor those coming off i.v. drugs, where possible, to test them for sero-positivity and to advise them on safe sex guidelines.

Medical Injuries

The most obvious example of a medical injury in which care staff are exposed to possible infection is the needle-stick injury. In practice, the risk of infection appears low. Other medical procedures also apparently carry a low risk. There has not been a single case of a health professional developing AIDS purely as a result of his or her work. Nonetheless, there is at least a theoretical risk. Patients should be advised to inform their doctor before any invasive procedure is undertaken, so that appropriate precautions can be taken. Similar considerations apply to dentists, since most dental procedures involve some exposure to blood. Further details on the risks of medical procedures are reviewed in Chapter 3.

Tattooing and Other Cosmetic Procedures

Tattooing is theoretically a way of transmitting the virus much as it can be transmitted by needle sharing. This is likely to be the case where the tattooist uses the same needle on more than one person or where more than one person at a time is tattooed. It may be difficult for the average tattooist to adequately sterilise equipment, and the use of disposable needles is the only safe approach. Sero-positives should not be tattooed.

It is possible that other procedures may cause a risk. Being shaved in the barber's is a theoretical risk and patients should be advised to avoid it. Ear piercing may also present a risk. Most people doing ear piercing professionally use disposable needles, but a fair amount of ear piercing seems to be an amateur business done by friends, with poor hygiene.

Giving of Blood and Donation of Organs

Clearly, patients in high-risk groups should donate neither blood nor organs. Many people carry organ donor cards in their wallets, which they have forgotten about. These cards should be destroyed by sero-positives. In the same way, they should not give semen.

Sharing of Toothbrushes and Razors with Others in the Home

Toothbrushes and razors may be contaminated with blood.

Miscellaneous

Any procedure in which blood can be transmitted can present a risk of AIDS — for example, 'blood brotherhood rites', biting a partner during sex and drawing blood, and so on. There are many possibilities. However, these are never likely to prove major transmission routes for HTLV-III. Provided that patients are aware of the way in which the virus is passed on, they can exercise common-sense to avoid the risk of transmission.

THINGS WHICH ARE NOT A RISK

It is often as useful for a patient to know what is not a risk as to know what is a risk. Clearly, the HTLV-III virus is not particularly infectious except through the routes outlined above. If it could be transmitted by casual contact, the pattern of cases would be very different from what is actually seen. It is worth listing what does not constitute a risk:

- HTLV-III cannot be transmitted by touching someone who has the virus, by being in the same room as them or by breathing the same air as them.

- HTLV-III is not transmitted by using restaurants or by drinking in bars.

- HTLV-III is not transmitted by sharing a house with someone or by hugging them or by kissing them on the cheek.

- HTLV-III is not transmitted by using the same WC or washbasin or bath as someone who is sero-positive.

In other words, there is no reason whatsoever why a sero-positive patient should not lead an entirely normal life. He or she is not a risk to family or friends or strangers. Media coverage would lead anyone to doubt this simple fact. It is therefore worth telling patients and their families specifically that this is the case. Even if they know the fact intellectually, it is often a great reassurance to actually hear someone who knows the facts tell them so.

Even where blood spillage takes place (after a patient suffers a cut with a knife, for instance), the risk is a small one. All that needs to be done is to clean surfaces with a 1:10 dilution of bleach. Further details of domestic management are contained in Chapter 6.

CONCLUSION

Clearly, with any set of risk-reduction procedures it is only possible to inform patients and to recommend steps they might take. Work at St Mary's suggests that where detailed information is provided to patients the great majority will take the necessary steps to reduce the risk of transmission (Green and Miller, in preparation). It seems clear that in this area, as in others, patients who are given the facts honestly and clearly and left to make their own decision will take those steps which protect both themselves and others.

REFERENCES

Barton, S. (1985). Personal communication

Bell, A. P. and Weinberg, M. S. (1978). *Homosexualities*. Mitchell Beazley, London

Cheingsong-Popov *et al.* (1984). Prevalence of antibodies to human t-lympho-tropic virus type III in AIDS and AIDS-risk patients in Britain. *Lancet*, **ii**, 477

Green, J. and Miller, D. (1985). In preparation

Jaffe, H. W., Choi, K., Thomas, P. A. *et al.* (1983). National case control study of Kaposi's Sarcoma and *Pneumocystis carinii* pneumonia in homosexual men: Part 1, Epidemiologic results. *Ann. Int. Med.*, **99**, 1983

Jones, P. (1985). *Aids and the Blood*. Haemophilia Society, London

Judson, F. N., Miller, K. G. and Schaffnit, T. R. (1977). Screening for gonorrhea and syphilis in the gay baths: Denver, Colorado. *Am. J. Pub. Hlth.*, **67**, 740

Marmor, M. (1984). Epidemic Kaposi's sarcoma and sexual practices in male homosexuals. In Friedman-Kein, A. (Ed.), *Progress in AIDS*. Masson, New York

Marmor, M., Friedman-Kein, A. E., Zolla-Pazner, S., Stahl, R. E. *et al.* (1984). Kaposi's Sarcoma in homosexual men: A seroepidemiological case-control study. *Ann. Int. Med.*, **100**, 809

Mulleady, G. and Green, J. (1985). In preparation

Murray-Sykes, K. (1983). Paper presented at Scientific Meeting, St. Mary's Hospital, London, October 1983

Ritchey, M. G. (1977). Venereal disease among homosexual men. *J. Am. Med. Assoc.*, **237**, 767

Saghir, M. T. and Robins, E. (1973). *Male and Female Homosexuality*. Williams and Wilkins, Baltimore

Sohn, N. and Bibilotti, J. G. (1977). The Gay Bowel Syndrome: A review of colonic and rectal conditions in 200 male homosexuals. *Am. J. Gastroenterol.*, **67**, 478

Roberts, T. (1985). In preparation

Weinberg, M. S. and Williams, C. J. (1974). *Male Homosexuals: Their Problems and Adaptation.* Oxford University Press, New York

Wright, R. and Wright, T. (1984). Living with AIDS. *Br. J. Sexual Med.*, **12**, 5

11
Hospital Counselling: Structure and Training

John Green and David Miller

STRUCTURE

Setting up a Counselling Service

The counselling of those with AIDS and AIDS-related problems is important for several reasons. First, AIDS is a sexually transmitted disease and someone infected with HTLV-III can pass it on to others. By informing and helping patients the risk of spread to others can be reduced. Second, there is evidence that the acquisition of intercurrent sexually transmitted diseases may provoke AIDS in those who are infected with the virus. If patients can be helped to make appropriate changes in life-style, they can sharply reduce their risk of intercurrent sexually transmitted diseases. Finally, AIDS causes considerable distress to patients and their families. Even those who are asymptomatic sero-positives often experience a high degree of psychological and social disturbance. Informed counselling can help to reduce the disturbance which patients experience and thus can relieve suffering, which is one of the major aims of all health care provision.

It is sometimes argued that setting up a counselling service costs money and that it must be justified in cost-effectiveness terms. Effective counselling can help to prevent the spread of the virus. It is only necessary to consider the cost of caring for AIDS patients, including tests, drugs, out-patient care and hospital admissions, to realise that if counsellors can help to prevent two or three new cases a year, they will have more than covered the cost of their salary.

Who Needs Counselling?

Five main groups of patients are likely to require counselling: (1) those with AIDS and AIDS-related complex (ARC); (2) those with PGL; (3) asymptomatic

HTLV-III sero-positives; (4) those who are concerned to reduce their risk of acquiring AIDS; (5) the lovers, families and friends of diagnosed patients. The discussion that follows is mainly concerned with out-patient counselling. Counselling of in-patients is covered in more detail below.

Personnel

In a real sense, everyone involved with a patient is likely to be involved in counselling him. However, it is very useful to have one or more people who will take responsibility for carrying out the bulk of the counselling work. This is important both from the point of view of ensuring that the work does, in fact, get done and because it allows a health district or hospital to identify personnel for training (see below).

Exactly who will carry the main role of AIDS counsellor will depend on the service in which they are working and on local circumstances. The majority of those involved in counselling patients, at least in the NHS in the UK, are likely to be working in, or closely with, genito-urinary medicine (GUM) clinics. However, similar principles apply to other services — for instance, haemophilia centres or the Blood Transfusion Service.

The counsellor needs certain skills:

- Knowledge about AIDS and the ability to keep up with a rapidly developing field.
- Basic counselling skills.
- The ability to work with a wide range of other professionals and to communicate clearly with them.
- The ability to recognise patients who need more specialised referral — for instance, those who have become very depressed.

Most of these skills can be developed with appropriate training (see below). However, some experience in counselling others is clearly an advantage. This is not the same thing as having a formal counselling qualification. Many professional counselling courses teach skills which confer little advantage in this context. Some schools of counselling use approaches in which the counsellor is trained not to give advice, clearly a disadvantage in this field.

The most obvious person to carry out counselling is the doctor carrying out treatment of a case. However, in most settings this is simply out of the question because of the lack of individual patient time. Nor do all doctors necessarily have the aptitude or inclination to carry out such work. However, it is helpful if medical staff dealing with patients with AIDS-related problems play some part in counselling where possible.

In some hospitals psychiatrists or clinical psychologists may play a large part in counselling. They will usually have relevant experience in working with those who are very distressed. Even where they do carry out the bulk of counselling, it is helpful to be able to refer particular cases to psychologists or psychiatrists. However, again, lack of manpower and time are likely to prove a problem.

In most GUM clinics the health advisor or clinic nurse is likely to be the main counsellor. AIDS counselling is a natural extension of their role in other sexually transmitted diseases. AIDS is a rather different disease from other sexually transmitted diseases in that it is potentially fatal and, at the moment, incurable. Therefore, it calls for somewhat different skills from the counselling of those with, say, syphilis or gonorrhoea. Nonetheless, familiarity with sexually transmitted disease counselling and GUM clinic procedures forms a valuable base on which to build up the necessary skills.

In a busy urban GUM or BTS clinic a full-time AIDS counsellor, and sometimes more than one, will be required. In areas where there are few AIDS cases and few sero-positives the work might form only part of the duties of the counsellor.

Setting up a System

It is clearly a waste of time having a counsellor if the patients do not get to see him or her. Unless there is a clear system, understood by everyone, that is exactly what will happen.

The first step is to pre-counsel those coming in for the test. They must consider whether they want the test in the light of possible implications in terms of insurance (and, e.g., mortgages), employment and other issues. In most GUM clinics patients will turn up at any time during clinic hours and their reason for attendance will not be known in advance. Most clinics are likely to find it difficult to allot a counsellor simply to stand by in case a patient should appear who needs pre-counselling. If a patient cannot be pre-counselled at the time of arrival, he can always be offered a fixed appointment later. The provision of some written material on the HTLV-III antibody test, its meaning and possible consequences, and ways of reducing risk is well worth while when a patient comes in for the first time for testing.

Most counselling is likely to be done when test results are known. The most sensible way to handle this is for the doctor to give a definite appointment for the patient to return to get his or her results. This can be arranged so that the counsellor is available to see the patient immediately after he or she is told the results.

It is well worth counselling sero-negatives as well as sero-positives. Sero-negatives seeking to establish their HTLV-III status are clearly concerned about the risk and are usually very receptive to sensible advice.

It is important that the counsellor should have all the available information on a patient. Counselling someone with ARC is likely to be rather different from counselling someone with PGL and not other symptoms.

Also, if a patient is being seen repeatedly over a period of time, it is vital that the counsellor have information on his or her current health and any changes in this.

Where AIDS patients or those with ARC are involved, it is useful for everyone involved with cases to meet from time to time for an 'out-patient round'. This is particularly important because so many different departments tend to be involved with each patient because of the range of problems shown.

Not infrequently several different hospitals and community services are involved in the care of a patient. Under these circumstances the counsellor can play a useful role in keeping in touch with the various parties involved. Patients under the care of several hospitals or several departments within a hospital are frequently confused. This situation is worsened if each hospital or department sees it as someone else's responsibility to provide the pateint with information about his or her overall condition.

Another source of difficulty is where different staff involved in the care of a patient give different information. For many reasons, this situation occurs not infrequently.

It is vital that everyone should know what everyone else has said to a patient and have a rough idea what they are going to tell the patient in the future. In one case known to the authors a patient was being seen by more than one hospital and there was a considerable delay in informing him that AIDS had been confirmed, simply because everyone thought someone else had told him.

Offering conflicting information and advice is a particular problem in counselling. As noted above, many of the staff involved with a patient are carrying out a certain amount of counselling with the patient. However, it is vital that one person — the counsellor or some other agreed person — should co-ordinate the main part of the counselling. To have several people, all of whom think they are 'counselling' the patient, is a recipe for disaster and will usually leave an unhappy and confused patient, particularly if everyone is taking a different approach. As in every other area of health care, it is important that everyone should be clear about their roles at the outset. A schematic analysis of possible counselling referral and liaison procedures is presented in Figure 11.1.

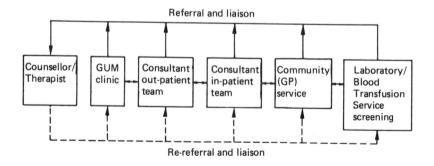

Figure 11.1 Possible counselling referral and liaison procedure

Counselling In-patients

Many AIDS patients are diagnosed, not in the GUM clinic but as in-patients in a hospital ward. It is vital that the counsellor should be introduced as early as possible to the patient, preferably soon after the patient has been told the diagnosis. It is also important that the counsellor should be introduced as a normal part of the clinical team, particularly if he or she is a psychologist or a psychiatrist. Some patients will see a visit by someone from these professions as a sign that they are thought to be mentally ill if the introduction is mishandled.

With in-patients, ward staff, especially nursing staff, play a key role. They are with the patient most of the time. Consequently, it is to them that patients will often turn. Any AIDS counsellor must recognise the vital importance of this role and must co-operate with nursing staff to ensure that the patient receives the best support possible. Not only patients turn to ward nursing staff. Relatives, also, seek information and support from ward staff. They also ask difficult and often upsetting questions. Some relatives react with anger to finding that their loved one has AIDS, and may turn this anger on those who have made the diagnosis and are providing essential care.

Working with AIDS patients can be very stressful. Few hospital staff find it easy to deal with young people who are dying. It is often helpful, where large numbers of patients are being seen, for there to be a support group for staff with whom they can talk over the problems. It is a mistake to try to force such meetings into a deep exploration of feelings. Most people do not want or require such solemn discussions. But it can be helpful to have a meeting at which people can admit how they do feel and find out, inevitably, that others feel the same things. They may also, via such meetings, model and develop their own effective management and coping skills, perhaps by a temporary reallocation of duties in cases of conspicuous staff stress.

Support Groups for Patients

AIDS patients and sero-positives often gain considerably from the experiences of others. They are able to share difficulties they are having and also to hear the ways in which others have dealt with their difficulties. Where a clinic has a number of patients in the same group, it is worth while forming a support group. It is important for the counsellor to be there — at least initially — and to be available to attend when necessary.

Fortnightly evening meetings are the most useful format. It is helpful to have two people leading the group — initially, at least. It is, of course, important to find a comfortable, private room in which to hold meetings. Again, it is not necessary to force the groups into any particular format. They need not be aimed at uncovering people's deepest feelings (although these sometimes do appropriately emerge and undergo sharing and discussion). Often it is practical coping issues which patients want most to discuss, and a support group fulfils important social needs as well, providing a context in which the common diagnosis can be discussed without fear of 'discovery' or intolerance and fearful isolation can be overcome.

Ideally the group will take on the organising and running of its own meetings eventually.

TRAINING

Experience has taught that effective post-diagnostic management needs, above all, consistency. This consistency must be reflected in the allocation of particular treatment roles to particular individuals (avoiding duplication and confusion) and in the nature of information given to particular patients (and the emphasis of that information). It should also go without saying that a certain 'quality control' is very necessary in counselling, so that the quality of counselling intervention is maintained across individuals, departments and hospitals. Providing the best possible intervention for the care of all patients must be the top priority. Particularly in this context, a consistent approach in counselling (e.g. regarding risk reduction) is of the utmost importance, given that the correct advice may save lives.

From this perspective, the authors have developed a counselling training programme for all hospital staff (doctors, psychologists, nurses, health advisors, social workers, etc.) that emphasises consistency and quality control. The training is in the format of a 2 day 'workshop' featuring input on clinical diagnosis and management, together with a wide range of counselling issues, role plays and paper-case discussion (topics are listed in Table 11.1). Although a longer programme is, in the authors' view, desirable, the pressure of numbers makes this difficult. The usually wide patient-contact experience of participants renders the need for this less urgent than the need for briefer training. It is made clear to participants, however, that the counselling training workshop is designed to equip health professionals with an understanding of the needs of patients and those affected by diagnosis, and with some resources for meeting these needs. It is not a form of qualification for the task.

The topics covered will not be discussed in detail, as they form the substance of this book! It has been found useful to reinforce each presentation with detailed written summaries, so that lessons learnt are not forgotten owing to participant overload! Familiarisation with essential and practical counselling issues is boosted by rehearsing the problem-solving and other counselling strategies using paper-case material based on actual experiences (patient anonymity is strenuously assured prior to material preparation). In order to make this easier, participants are divided into groups of five people, each having responsibility for drawing up counselling and problem-solving strategies for two particular cases. Feedback and discussion is then obtained from all the participants.

Table 11.1   Counselling training 'workshop' format

Day 1

Current medical knowledge and future developments. Epidemiology, clinical diagnosis and manifestations, medical treatments, etc.

Homosexual life-styles and sexuality, and haemophilia. Research and anecdotal evidence, the impact of AIDS, resulting problems

Introduction to AIDS counselling. Range of counselling issues, experiences and tactics

Breaking bad news. How to inform patients, lovers and relatives of diagnoses, and resulting management issues

Counselling and support of the terminally ill. Experiences and tactics from cancer care and hospice management

Day 2

HTLV-III and PGL counselling in risk reduction and safer sex. Risk reduction, health boosting, and safer sex for all risk groups

Practical counselling management. Basic counselling methodology, experiences and tactics. Problem solving with practice and feedback

Helping partners and relatives. Management and support of lovers and families of all patient groups

Diagnosis and treatment of anxiety. Signs, symptoms, differential diagnosis and treatment. The significance of anxiety in AIDS and AIDS-related disorders

Diagnosis and treatment of depression and obsessional disorders. Signs, symptoms, differential diagnosis and treatment. The significance of depression and obsessional disorders in patient groups. The management of suicide and of those at risk

Paper-case analysis. Small-group analysis and discussion, role plays and feedback

---

The format of each workshop varies according to the specialties represented by the participants. For instance, BTS personnel will require less AIDS discussion than staff from haemophilia centres or infectious diseases wards.

It is envisaged that every health district in the UK will have at least one or two persons with experience of this course, in order to be able to provide the necessary planning and training for their own staff when and if AIDS becomes a relevant management issue in their district. In this way, an effective counselling structure can be created to meet the particular needs of each health district and service. Key staff will be identified, and effective liaison will be made between hospitals and appropriate community counselling and support agencies. In this way, a relevant and cost-effective system will, it is hoped, be established in time to meet future requirements from overlapping disciplines.

Appendix: Useful Addresses for High-risk Groups

Body Positive. A resource and support organisation for those who are HTLV-III sero-positive.
Address: Body Positive, BM Aids, London WC1N 3XX

The Terrence Higgins Trust. A registered charity providing face-to-face and telephone counselling, support groups and 'buddy' services for those with AIDS, and an information service for those with AIDS-related worries.
Address: Terrence Higgins Trust, BM AIDS, London WC1N 3XX
Telephone Help Line: 01-278 8745 (8.00-10.00 p.m., Mon.-Fri.)

London Gay Switchboard. A telephone advisory, counselling and referral service for gay people and for those with health-related concerns, run completely by gay people.
Telephone: 01-837 7324 (24 hours daily, year round)

Haemophilia Society. Information, research and advisory service for haemophiliacs and their families.
Address: PO Box 9, 16 Trinity Street, London SE1 1DE
Telephone: 01-407 1010

Health Education Council
Address: 78 Oxford Street, London WC1A 1AH
Telephone: 01-631 0930

Index